Women and Social Policy
An introduction

edited by

Christine Hallett

Professor of Social Policy
University of Stirling

PRENTICE HALL
HARVESTER WHEATSHEAF

LONDON   NEW YORK   TORONTO   SYDNEY   TOKYO   SINGAPORE
MADRID   MEXICO CITY   MUNICH

in association with

THE SOCIAL POLICY ASSOCIATION
WOMEN AND SOCIAL POLICY GROUP

First published 1996 by
Prentice Hall Europe
Campus 400, Maylands Avenue
Hemel Hempstead
Hertfordshire HP2 7EZ
A division of
Simon & Schuster International Group

Typeset in 10/12pt Ehrhardt
by Dorwyn Ltd, Rowlands Castle, Hants

Printed and bound in Great Britain
by T.J. Press (Padstow) Ltd

Library of Congress Cataloging in Publication Data

Women and social policy: an introduction/edited by Christine
  Hallett.
      p.   cm.
    Includes bibliographical references (p.   ) and index.
    ISBN 0–13–353889–3 (pbk.)
      1. Women social workers – Great Britain.   2. Social work with
  women – Great Britain.   I. Hallett, Christine.
  HV40.46.W65   1995
  362.83′0941–dc20
                                                      95–22968
                                                          CIP

British Library Cataloguing in Publication Data

A catalogue record for this book is available
from the British Library

ISBN 0–13–353889–3 (pbk)

    3   4   5   00   99   98   97

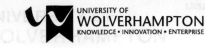

Contents

Figures

Tables

Contributors

Claire Callender is a Senior Fellow at the Policy Studies Institute, London. Previously she worked for the Institute of Employment Studies (formerly the Institute of Manpower Studies) (1989–94) and as a lecturer at the Universities of Cardiff, Leeds and Bradford (1979–88). Her research has focused on women and the labour market and especially issues concerning employment, training and social security policies. She has written widely in these areas. She is currently conducting research on the personal and financial consequences of the failure of small firms and is continuing her research on NVQs.

Ann Davis is Director of Social Work Research and Development at the University of Birmingham. She teaches, researches and publishes in the fields of gender, users' views, poverty and social work. Her recent publications include co-authorship of a report on user involvement in European public welfare services and a book *Poverty-aware Social Work* (Arena, 1996).

Rosemary Deem is Professor of Educational Research and Dean of the Faculty of Social Sciences at Lancaster University and currently Chairperson of the British Sociological Association. She has been working on gender issues in education since the mid-1970s and her publications include *Women and Schooling* (1978), *Schooling for Women's Work* (1980) and (ed.) *Co-education Reconsidered* (1984). During most of the 1980s she was a Labour County Councillor in Buckinghamshire and also Chair of

Governors at Stantonbury Campus Comprehensive in Milton Keynes. From 1990 until 1993 she co-directed an Economic and Social Research Council funded study on the reforms of school governance in England, with Dr Kevin J. Brehony of the University of Reading, and is now writing a book, *Active Citizenship and the Governing of Schools* with Dr Brehony and Suzanne Heath. Work has just begun on a new project about women and holidays with Dr Penny Tinkler of Manchester University.

Peggy Foster is a lecturer in social policy at the University of Manchester. She is co-author with J. Dale of *Feminists and State Welfare* (Routledge and Kegan Paul, 1986) and author of *Women and the Health Care Industry: An unhealthy relationship?* (Open University Press, 1995).

Christine Hallett is Professor of Social Policy and Head of the Department of Applied Social Science at the University of Stirling. She has previously taught at the Universities of Keele, Western Australia and Leicester. She has researched and written widely on the topics of child protection and the personal social services. Publications include *Women and Social Services Departments* (Harvester Wheatsheaf, 1989) and *Interagency Co-ordination in Child Protection: A case study* (HMSO, 1995).

Carol-Ann Hooper is a lecturer in social policy at the University of York. She is the author of *Mothers Surviving Child Sexual Abuse* (Routledge, 1992) and of several articles on men's violence to women and children.

Margaret May and Edward Brunsdon teach social policy at London Guildhall University. Their recent publications include articles on welfare provision in Sweden and employer care. They are currently researching private welfare in Britain and Sweden.

Jane Millar is Professor of Social Policy at the University of Bath. Her main area of research interest is in the relationship between the state, the family and the labour market in determining access to resources and living standards. She has written widely on the topic of women and poverty including editing, with Caroline Glendinning, *Women and Poverty in Britain*, and *Women and Poverty in Britain: The 1990s*, both published by Harvester Wheatsheaf, 1987 and 1992 respectively. The circumstances of lone-parent families and the nature of the state support they receive are another area of interest, and with Jonathan Bradshaw she was responsible for carrying out the first national UK survey of these families (J. Bradshaw and J. Millar, *Lone-Parent Families in the UK*, HMSO, 1991). Her current research includes a comparative study of the way in which family obligations are defined in policy in the member states of the European Union.

Shafquat Nasir is a lecturer in social policy at Manchester Metropolitan University. She has worked in a number of women's projects around issues of domestic violence and child sexual abuse, and has been involved in refuge work, research and policy development. She returned to education at the Manchester Metropolitan University, where she was later appointed as lecturer in social policy. She also does some teaching at Bradford University and is currently involved in consultancy work for two projects, one related to Black people, HIV and AIDS and the other to homelessness amongst young lesbians and gay men.

Susan Tester has an extensive background in social research and was formerly based in London at the Centre for Policy on Ageing, the Policy Studies Institute, and the London School of Economics. She is currently a lecturer in social policy at the University of Stirling, where she specialises in community care, ageing and comparative social policy. Recent publications include *Community Care for Older People: A comparative perspective* (Macmillan, 1995).

Roberta Woods has worked in local government and for a number of years taught housing management/policy at the Universities of Ulster and Newcastle. She currently teaches at Ruskin College, Oxford. She has written on various social security and housing issues and is currently undertaking a major research project on women's access to local authority housing.

Preface

This volume has its origins in a meeting of the Women and Social Policy Group of the Social Policy Association chaired by Dr Dulcie Groves at the SPA's Annual Conference held at the University of Nottingham in July 1992. Several of the women present noted that the pioneering texts on women and welfare (such as Ungerson, 1985; Dale and Foster, 1986; Pascall, 1986; Williams, 1989) which had served us well in the 1980s were in need of revision to take account of developments in both feminist theory and social policy. Later we learned that there were to be new editions of some of these key texts. However, a decision was also taken at the meeting to produce a new volume on women and social policy. Clare Grist of Harvester Wheatsheaf, who was present at the meeting, subsequently commissioned the volume which was publicised in the SPA Newsletter with a call for contributions. The SPA Executive Committee endorsed the initiative, resulting in the publication of this book by Harvester Wheatsheaf in association with the SPA.

As is clear in the succeeding chapters, the recognition of the gendered nature of the relations involved in the production and consumption of social welfare has been a key development in the analysis of social policy in recent years. This volume examines the position and experiences of women as users and providers of social welfare in a range of settings, formal and informal, in the mixed economy of welfare. It emphasises the difference and diversity amongst women which shape the specificity of their lives as their experience varies and identities shift through the life course, for example, as older women, Black women, mothers, carers, lesbians or as women with disabilities.

xvi *Preface*

However the volume also recognises the systematic and apparently enduring gendered patterning and inequalities in social policy which have persisted throughout almost forty years of the 'welfare state'.

As editor, I am grateful to Clare Grist of Harvester Wheatsheaf for her encouragement, support and patience in the production of this volume and to the contributing authors, without whom it would not have been possible. I am also grateful to colleagues at the University of Stirling: to Sue Dyer, Lynsey Hill and Sally Armstrong-Payne for secretarial help; to Alison Giles, Computing Adviser, for help in preparing the composite list of references; and to Sue Scott, Cathy Taylor and Sue Tester for their comments and advice. Finally, I acknowledge, with gratitude, the support of the Women and Social Policy Group and the Executive Committee of the Social Policy Association.

1   *Social policy: continuities and change*

Christine Hallett

The term 'social policy' is used in two principal ways – both as the name of an academic discipline (or, as some would argue, a field or focus of study) and as a description of the societal arrangements for the provision of social welfare. This chapter outlines the nature of social policy in both senses, reviewing briefly some of the key characteristics of social policy as a subject of study and of social policies, as they exist in the United Kingdom, to provide a context for the detailed consideration of specific policy domains and issues in subsequent chapters.

The scope of social policy

It is not easy to define the term 'social policy'. In part, this is because there have been important changes in the discipline in recent years expanding its concerns beyond social administration, but also because it is difficult clearly to delineate social policy from economic or other types of public policy. While defence policy is normally considered to be distinct from social policy, there are social consequences of, for example, frequent service moves in terms of family welfare, or of the economic restructuring required in the defence industry, following the changes resulting from the ending of the so-called cold war. Similarly, transport and environmental policy can have important consequences for social welfare but they have not traditionally been encompassed within the central concerns of social policy. More recently, however, these areas have engaged the attention of social policy analysts. In respect of transport, for example, Le Grand (1982) and Beuret (1991) discuss its redistributional consequences in terms respectively of social class and gender. In the early 1990s, social policy analysts also embraced environmental policy issues (see e.g. Cahill, 1991; Ferris, 1991; Pierson, 1991; Wilding, 1992; George and Wilding, 1994). Perhaps most important of all, there are continuing debates (discussed by Callender in Chapter 3) concerning the relationship between employment and social policy.

Despite the definitional difficulties at the boundaries, there is broad consensus over the core concerns of social policy. They are the societal arrangements made for the provision of welfare in four key areas of housing, education, health and income maintenance or social security. A fifth form of service provision is conventionally added to the list, namely the personal social services. (These are the services of advice and advocacy, care and control provided in residential, day and domiciliary settings to children and families, older people and people with a physical or mental disability by staff of local authority social services departments and the private and voluntary sectors.) In the United Kingdom there is a strong, although by no means exclusive, tradition of state provision in each of these five areas. These services are at the core of the welfare state.

State welfare

One trend of fundamental importance in the United Kingdom (and in other so-called developed countries) in the past 100 years has been the vast increase in the scope and range of state activity. This is reflected in the growth in the proportion of the nation's wealth which is devoted to public expenditure and, of particular importance for social policy analysts, the rise in the proportion of spending devoted to social welfare. As Table 1.1 illustrates, while total government spending increased from 12.7 to 57.9 per cent of GNP between 1910 and 1975 (a roughly five-fold increase), social welfare spending increased approximately seven-fold from 4.2 per cent of GNP to 28.8 per cent. Figure 1.1 shows that social service spending has remained at similar levels in the succeeding fifteen years to 1990.

Throughout this century, as Figure 1.1 illustrates, the overall trend has been upward, accompanied by bursts of activity associated with particular historical circumstances. One such was the package of liberal welfare reforms following the turn of the century, including the introduction of school meals in 1906, old-age pensions in 1909 and the National Insurance Act 1911. Another, often labelled the period of the 'creation' of the welfare state, occurred in the 1940s as plans for reconstruction developed during the Second World War were implemented in a succession of legislative measures. Among the most important were the arrangements for social security introduced by the Family Allowances and the National Insurance Acts in 1946 and the National Assistance Act 1948 following the Beveridge Report on *Social*

Table 1.1 The growth of social expenditure in the United Kingdom

	Percentage of GNP at factor cost							
	1910	1921	1931	1937	1951	1961	1971	1975
All social services	4.2	10.1	12.7	10.9	16.1	17.6	23.8	28.8
Social security		4.7	6.7	5.2	5.3	6.7	8.9	9.5
Welfare		1.1	1.8	1.8	4.5	0.3	0.7	1.1
Health						4.1	5.1	6.0
Education		2.2	2.8	2.6	3.2	4.2	6.5	7.6
Housing		2.1	1.3	1.4	3.1	2.3	2.6	4.6
Infrastructure	0.7	0.6	1.0	1.0	3.6	4.8	6.3	6.8
Industry	1.8	4.5	3.2	2.8	6.9	4.9	6.5	8.3
Justice and law	0.6	0.8	0.8	0.7	0.6	0.8	1.3	1.5
Military	3.5	5.6	2.8	5.0	10.8	7.6	6.6	6.2
Debt interest and other	1.9	7.7	8.2	5.2	6.9	6.3	5.9	6.3
Total state expenditure	12.7	29.4	28.8	25.7	44.9	42.1	50.3	57.9
Total state revenue	11.0	24.4	25.0	23.8	42.7	38.5	48.6	46.6
Borrowing requirement	1.7	5.0	3.8	1.9	2.2	3.6	1.7	11.3

Source: Gough (1979:77)

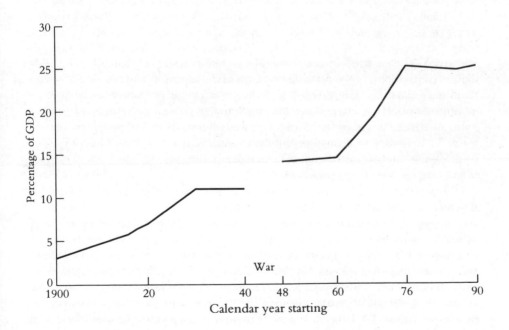
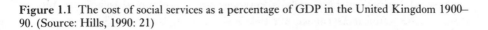

Figure 1.1 The cost of social services as a percentage of GDP in the United Kingdom 1900–90. (Source: Hills, 1990: 21)

Insurance and Allied Services, published in 1942; the introduction of a National Health Service in 1948 and the reform of education enshrined in the Education Act, 1944.

The welfare state constituted a commitment which modified the play of market forces (Wedderburn, 1965). It redrew the lines between public and private, between individualism and collectivism, and between the state, the market and the family as sources of social welfare. In the process as Marshall (1994: 133) notes 'distinctly gendered roles of citizen, worker and client begin to emerge as shaping the relationship of the state to its populace'. The purposes, functioning and outcomes of these areas of state activity have been, and remain, of central concern to social policy analysts. As Wilding (1992) notes, the growth of social policy as a subject of study accompanied the rise in state welfare from the 1950s to the 1970s.

The mixed economy of welfare

Notwithstanding the importance of conventionally defined social services in social policy, in a seminal article entitled 'The social division of welfare' Titmuss (1958) drew attention to other sources of supply of social welfare. Titmuss argued that it was important for social policy analysts to study the welfare functions performed by varied social arrangements rather than to restrict the focus to particular institutions. In addition to state-provided social welfare, he identified two other important mechanisms for the redistribution of resources in the pursuit of welfare objectives, namely fiscal and occupational welfare. Fiscal welfare comprises welfare provided through the taxation system. In so far as allowances are granted against tax liability to individuals or corporations, the government may be said to be incurring tax expenditures. Significant allowances are granted to individuals in the pursuit of social welfare objectives, notably the married persons' tax allowance, constituting, in effect, a government subsidy to a particular form of household formation, and mortgage interest tax relief, a subsidy to people buying their home with a mortgage. Other types of fiscal welfare include tax allowances for older people for the purchase of private health care and the blind persons' allowance.

Occupational welfare, as the name implies, refers to welfare services or benefits to which entitlement derives from paid employment. Most significant among these are occupational pensions, although access to services such as company housing, subsidised education and private health care and maternity pay and leave are also included. Labour market experiences differ widely in respect of both ethnicity and gender in matters such as pay, continuities and discontinuities in employment and hours of work. In consequence, women, Black and White, are generally less privileged recipients of occupational welfare than men, particularly in respect of pensions (Groves, 1992) but also more broadly, as May and Brunsdon discuss in Chapter 11.

Titmuss thus identified two important sources of welfare supply beyond state social welfare provision in the social division of welfare. Of all three he wrote:

When we examine them in turn, it emerges that this division is not based on any fundamental difference in the functions of the three systems . . . or their declared aims. . . . So far as the ultimate aims of these systems are concerned, it is argued that their similarities are more important than their dissimilarities. The definition for most purposes of what is a 'social service' should take its stand on aims: not on the administrative methods and institutional devices employed to achieve them. (Titmuss, 1958: 42)

Subsequent analysts have added to the list of components of a pluralistic welfare system, identifying private markets, voluntary social services and the informal sector of family and community as constituting with the three outlined above the key providers in the mixed economy of welfare. These varied sources of supply are examined in subsequent chapters of this book, a central theme of which is that the mixed economy of welfare embodies gendered assumptions, operates in gendered ways and has gendered redistributional effects.

The end of consensus

The changes in the welfare mix (which have had important consequences for won en as users and providers of social welfare) were linked with major debates about th future of welfare. It is widely accepted that in Britain following the Second World War there was a degree of cross-party and wider societal consensus about the provision of social welfare and, in particular, the role of the welfare state. An endorsement of the universalist principles adopted in the 1940s was seen in both the Labour and Conservative parties in the 1950s and 1960s and epitomised by the term 'Butskellism' – an amalgam of the names of the Tory leader R.A. Butler and the Labour leader Hugh Gaitskell. The discipline of social policy developed alongside the growth in state welfare, and it too was said to be dominated by a reformist, empiricist, social democratic/Fabian socialist consensus.

It may be argued that the emphasis on consensus during this period both in the politics of welfare and in the discipline of social policy has been exaggerated (Johnson, 1987; Bulmer *et al.*, 1989). For example, the right-wing think tank, the Institute of Economic Affairs, produced pamphlets on social welfare during this period (e.g. Seldon, 1957), Friedman published *Capitalism and Freedom* in 1962, and it is clear from Titmuss' writings (e.g. Titmuss, 1968) that social policy students were exposed to the debates concerning choices and markets in welfare. In 1958, for example, Titmuss reviewed writing about the welfare state since 1948 and concluded that the dominant note was that it was established too quickly and on too broad a scale and that, in consequence, it had been harmful to the economic health of the nation and its 'moral fibre' (Titmuss, 1958: 35). From a different perspective, Saville (1957/8) outlined a neo–Marxist explanation of the welfare state, pointing to the combined role of working-class struggle, state action to pre-empt more radical demands and the needs and interests of the capitalist state in accounting for historical developments. None the less, the relative certainties and orthodoxies of the post-war years do contrast sharply with the more polarised debates over social welfare associated with the recession, the rise in oil prices, and inflation in the economic crisis of the mid-1970s.

The challenge to the social democratic consensus was posed by the New Right and by neo-Marxist analyses. From different points of origin, both postulated a link between the performance of the economy and the rising costs of welfare. The left, particularly in the work of O'Connor (1973) and Gough (1979), argued that the pursuit of the core functions of the capitalist state (namely, securing the conditions for capital accumulation and for legitimation) led to a fiscal crisis as government spending outstripped revenue. The New Right pointed to the alleged harmful economic consequences of state welfare programmes in diverting funds from investment, fostering a large unproductive human service workforce, inducing dependency and undermining work incentives. Both neo-Marxist and New Right critiques of social welfare arrangements also identified the relations of consumption as problematic – particularly, the unresponsiveness of state welfare bureaucracies and the power of professional providers over consumers. For the New Right, this was framed largely in terms of denial of individual freedom and choice, while neo-Marxists emphasised social control and oppression.

Despite some similarities in their analyses of existing welfare provision, the two ideological perspectives had fundamentally different starting points. The New Right, adopting and adapting free-market liberal ideas, emphasised individual freedom, choice and the supremacy of markets as a distributional mechanism and combined these with a cultural conservatism, based on respect for traditional sources of authority including the family and the Church, and populism (Pierson, 1991). The Marxists stressed that capitalism was antithetical to welfare and they emphasised equality and collective provision to meet social need. The policy prescriptions which followed (although much more fully articulated by the New Right) were very different. The significance was that the orthodoxies were challenged as social welfare was hotly debated in politics, popular opinion and in the discipline of social policy. (For fuller accounts of these developments see, for example Mishra, 1977, 1984; Glennerster and Midgley, 1991; Pierson, 1991; George and Wilding, 1994.)

Alongside the rise in contested views concerning the political economy of welfare, critiques of existing provision extended the analysis beyond social class to other groups. Class is a central analytic category in Marxism and a concern with poverty has been an enduring feature of social policy analysis since the nineteenth century. In the late 1970s and 1980s, however, attention also came to be paid to other social divisions and their implications for social policy, with a focus upon older people (see e.g. Sontag, 1978; Phillipson, 1982; Norman, 1985; Townsend, 1986; Featherstone and Hepworth, 1989), people with disabilities (Oliver, 1990; Morris, 1991–92), the welfare experiences of gays and lesbians (see e.g. Hart and Richardson, 1981; Anlin, 1989) and people from minority ethnic communities (see e.g. Brown, 1984; Bryan *et al.*, 1985; Norman, 1985; Gordon, 1986; Williams, 1987, 1989; Bhat *et al.*, 1988). In respect of minority ethnic groups, Williams (1989) demonstrated the salience of the themes of race and nation and the legacy of British imperialism in the development of domestic social policies. *Inter alia*, these writers explored the ways in which the needs of different groups were constructed, the assumptions upon which policies were developed, differential access to services was gained and differential impacts for service users resulted.

Feminist perspectives

Gender was, perhaps, the key social division which came to renewed prominence at this time. The rise of feminist perspectives on social welfare, associated with second-wave feminism from the late 1960s onwards, is central to this book. As Williams notes:

> Between the publication in 1977 of Elizabeth Wilson's *Women and the Welfare State* and Jen Dale and Peggy Foster's *Feminists and State Welfare* and Gillian Pascall's *Social Policy: A feminist analysis* in 1986, a wealth of material from different feminist perspectives emerged about the relationship between the state and the family, and about the financial, emotional and physical relationships within and outside the family. Much of this work offered new dimensions to key questions in social policy analysis; issues of caring, dependency, needs, of the relationship between work and income, of the relationships between the providers and users of welfare provision, as well as theoretical questions about the relationship between patriarchy, capitalism and the state. (Williams, 1989: xii)

The feminist analyses drew on different traditions, which were classified as liberal feminism, radical feminism and socialist feminism by Dale and Foster (1986), as radical feminism, Marxist feminism, liberalism and dual-systems theory by Walby (1990b), and as libertarian feminism, liberal feminism, welfare feminism, radical feminism, socialist feminism and Black feminism by Williams (1989). All the perspectives reflect an awareness of the structural subordination and oppression of women and the view that 'women's subordination must be questioned and challenged' (Abbott and Wallace, 1990: 10). However, they differ in their analysis of its causes and in their proposals for political action and change. Stacey (1993) warns of the dangers of typologies of feminist theories which can exclude much feminist thinking, ignore complexities and contradictions within an individual's work and which run the risk of stereotyping feminist ideas. However, they are commonly used in social policy (and women's studies) texts (see e.g. Dale and Foster, 1986 and Williams, 1989). In the 1970s, the key differences were seen to be between liberal feminists, social feminists and radical feminists (Jaggar, 1983). Simplifying for the purposes of presentation here, liberal feminism had a concern with equal rights and equal access, for example, in education, employment and politics, accompanied by a belief in social reform, for example, equal-opportunities legislation as central to the advancement of women. By contrast, the two other key variants of feminist thought that were influential at that time theorised women's subordination in terms of social structure and social relations, whether capitalism or patriarchy. Marxist and socialist feminism consider gender inequality to derive from capitalism, in which 'class relations and the economic exploitation of one class by another are the central features of social structure and these determine the nature of gender relations' (Walby, 1990b: 4). The household is a key site of oppression with the reproduction of labour power (socially, in daily living, and biologically, across the generations) provided by the unpaid domestic labour of women. As George and Wilding suggest:

> [women's] unpaid labour in the home is a subsidy to capitalism because it reduces the cost of reproducing the next generation of workers and servicing male breadwinners. Women's assumed dependence in the family and on a male breadwinner depresses their own earning capacity because employers do not need to pay them the full cost of reproducing their own labour power. Their low pay reinforces women's dependency within marriage and on marriage – they need a share of men's earnings. . . . A symbiotic relationship therefore exists between capitalism and the family. (1994: 132)

Although the balance varies among Marxist and socialist feminists in the relative importance they accord to the material or the ideological, the role of capitalism in producing and reproducing gender inequality is central.

Radical feminism is often classified as being rooted in essentialist understandings of sex and gender, that is based on the assumption that gender differences are, like sex differences, biologically based and therefore manifest across time and space (see e.g. Segal's (1987) account in *Is the Future Female?*). While such readings of the work of writers such as Brownmiller (1976), Millett (1970), and Firestone (1974) are possible, if not inevitable, this construction of radical feminism in general belies much which is central to radical feminist work. Writers such as Delphy (1984), Walby (1990b), Jackson (1995) and Stacey (1993) rely on a non-essentialist theorisation of patriarchy which stresses both the primacy of gender relations and differences for social structure and social relations more generally, and also the materiality and the historical and cultural specificity of such relations. 'Patriarchal domination is not based upon pre-existing sex differences, rather gender exists as a social division because of patriarchal domination' (Jackson, 1995: 13). This materialist radical feminism has some salience for analysis of the relationship between women and the welfare state, for example Delphy's analysis of the patriarchal division of labour in the household (Delphy, 1984) and Pateman's understanding that the sexual contract undermines the possibility of women's access to equal citizenship (Pateman, 1988).

A common theme in feminist analysis at this time was a search for universal explanations of women's oppression, whether these were seen to lie in capitalism or in patriarchy or rooted in biological differences between men and women (Barrett and

Phillips, 1992). Subsequently, a powerful challenge to these universalising tendencies was mounted. As A. Phillips (1992: 211) notes:

> the first phase of the contemporary women's movement involved excited re-discovery of what women had in common, in recent years it is difference that has dominated the debate. . . . A feminism that focuses too exclusively on what seem to be similarities between women can pass over in silence the divisions by race and class.

The differences and divisions included those between working-class women, lesbians, women with disabilities and older women. However, it was the Black feminists who argued most cogently that White, often middle-class, feminists had failed to take account of the different histories and experiences of women from minority ethnic groups, for example, in the labour market and in the domestic sphere. As Walby notes:

> the best example of this is the debate on the family which has traditionally been seen by white feminist analysis as a major, if not the major, site of women's oppression by men . . . since the family is a site of resistance and solidarity against racism for women of colour, it does not hold the central place in account-ing for women's subordination that it does for white women. (1990b: 14)

See also Ramazanoglu, 1989 on this point. These writers (e.g. hooks, 1981; Carby, 1982; Amos and Parmar, 1984) emphasise diversity, difference and the historically, materially and culturally specific forms of oppression experienced by particular groups of women. These issues are explored further by Nasir in Chapter 2.

Postmodernity and social policy

The challenge posed by Black feminists to dominant forms of feminist theorising emphasised diversity and difference, the local and the specific in contast to universal and essentialist claims. They argued for a less uniform and more fragmented and contextualised view of women's position and experience. In this respect they chimed with broader contemporary developments in social theory, particularly those associated with postmodernism. However, in the main, Black feminists and others were arguing for the specific materiality of Black women's oppression whereas postmodernist theoris-ing pointed towards the disruption of all universalist categories, including 'race'.

Postmodernity is associated with the end of the grand ideologies or meta-narratives such as liberalism or Marxism, capitalism or patriarchy. Williams (1992: 205) sum-marises postmodernism as follows: 'put simply, the major shifts perceived to be taking place are from standardisation, uniformity and universalism to heterogeneity, fragmentation, diversity and difference.' In the context of massive social change and transformation in global capital and in industrial production, the universalising tend-

encies of the grand narratives are seen as unable to explain change or to serve as
guides to future action, particularly in the sphere of governance and politics. With
specific reference to social policy, Taylor-Gooby (1994: 385 and 399) notes:

> Postmodernism claims that the universalist themes of modern society (society-
> wide political ideologies, the nation–state, the theme of rational planning in
> government policy, the large-scale public or private sector bureaucracy) are
> obsolete, to be replaced by a plural interest in diversity and choice . . . the
> central theme is of deteriorating confidence in universalising approaches . . .
> and of increasing fragmentation and uncertainty in social life. These ap-
> proaches succeed in reflecting some of the principal developments in recent
> social policies – decentralisation, consumerism, the use of new technology to
> transform management, stress on the non-state sector, the decline in the status
> of professionals and experts and the growth of privatisation and individualism.

This questioning of the idea of progress, which is central to modernity and to the
process of social reform associated with the welfare state, poses a particular challenge
for a book of this kind which takes, as its starting point, the potential of social policy
to enhance welfare and the importance of analysing it from the standpoint of women
(while acknowledging, none the less, that all feminist standpoints are partial). Both
postmodernism and feminist theorising point to the dangers of a false essentialism
and universalism about the category 'women' and thus about women's needs, wants
and experiences of welfare.

Fundamental questions have been asked about how basic are the differences between
men and women and whether the category of gender can survive the postmodern
critique. As Di Stefano (1990: 65) suggests: 'on this view, gender is implicated in a
disastrous and oppressive fiction, the fiction of "women" which runs roughshod over
multiple differences among and within women who are ill-served by a conception of
gender as basic.' There is, however, a danger that the recognition and celebration of
diversity and difference, locality and specificity mask the communalities and structural
position(s) of women in contemporary British society. Taylor-Gooby has explored
similar issues in respect of economic liberalism. He suggests that 'economic liberalism is
the nearest approximation to a universal theme in world affairs' (1994: 388) with
consequences for social welfare in terms of financial constraints, privatisation, less
regulation in labour markets and increased inequality. He writes:

> If postmodernism denies the significance of such broad developments and
> substitutes a language of particularism and diversity, the approach may obscure
> one of the great reversals for the most vulnerable groups in a cloud of detail,
> may ignore the wood through enthusiasm for bark rubbing. (1994: 388–9)

In reflecting on whether it is legitimate to define 'women' as a social category distinct
from 'men' and to explore whether women have collective interests, Walby suggests
(1990b: 15–16):

the postmodern critics have made some valuable points about the potential dangers in theorising gender inequality at an abstract and general level. However, they go too far in denying the necessary impossibility and unproductive nature of such a project.

Nicholson (1990: 8) summarises the position as follows: 'to invoke the ideas of endless difference is for feminism either to self destruct or to finally accept an ontology of abstract individualism.' The volume is based on the premise that the effects of gender are basic in ways that we have yet to understand fully, that gender functions as a 'difference that makes a difference', even as it can no longer claim the legitimating mantle of *the* difference (Di Stefano, 1990: 78), and, with particular reference to social policy that 'while gender relations could potentially take an infinite number of forms, in actuality there are some widely repeated features' (Walby, 1990b: 16).

A key task, theoretically, is how to account for the oppression of women in both its 'endless variety and monotonous similarity' (Rubin, 1975, in Fraser and Nicholson, 1990: 28). Although the specific welfare experiences of women of different social class, ethnicity, sexual preference, disability and age may vary widely, there are structural factors constituting and affecting those experiences. Mayo and Weir (1993: 51) note that 'arguing the importance of acknowledging diversity is not at all the same as arguing that there are no key common interests which can be shared among feminists with fundamentally different perspectives.' In similar vein, Barrett and Phillips (1992: 9) conclude:

> the strategic questions that face contemporary feminism are now informed by a much richer understanding of heterogeneity and diversity; but they continue to revolve around the alliances, coalitions and commonalities that give meaning to the idea of feminism.

Central to this book are both the differences and commonalities experienced by women in relation to social welfare. Politically the commonalities may be important but the specificity of women's position, for example as an elderly Black woman, is also critical for individual women's lives at particular points and their experiences of social welfare.

Women and social welfare

In respect of social policy, Hernes (1987) has suggested that women have three major statuses: as service users, as providers and as participants in the political processes affecting social welfare. They may move in and out of these statuses at different points in the life course as varied experiences affect their identity. In respect of the first two, the position of women is primary. As service users, women's unequal participation and structural disadvantage in the labour market (discussed by

Callender in Chapter 3) lead to their over-representation amongst those in poverty and reliant on state support (discussed by Millar in Chapter 4) and to their relative disadvantages in the housing market (discussed by Woods in Chapter 5). As May and Brunsdon demonstrate in Chapter 11, women's relative poverty also limits their consumption of private welfare services. Furthermore, as Foster argues in Chapter 7, women in all their diversity are key consumers of health care, although not always on their own terms. Their socially constructed responsibilities for child-rearing, family health and caring also lead women to be the key points of contact – the brokers and negotiators – between family members and services, whether education, health care, social security, housing or the personal social services, and whatever the source of provision, statutory, private, voluntary or informal. Balbo (1987: 49) suggests:

> because many goods and services are provided outside the family by other institutions (firms, schools, hospitals and so on) and because access to them requires time and flexibility on the part of 'clients', someone has to do the work of dealing with these agencies, adapting to their often complex, time-consuming, rigid and bureaucratic procedures. It is women who keep in touch with teachers and school staff, who take children to clinics and hospitals, who visit welfare agencies to obtain the family's entitlement.

In so far as the sources of supply of welfare are fragmented, the task of co-ordinating and securing access to social welfare services is rendered more difficult.

Many women are also central as service providers in social welfare. In the informal sphere, the continued role of women in social reproduction places them at the heart of the provision of care within families, not only for dependent household members, such as children or adults with disabilities, as Tester demonstrates in Chapter 9, but also for able-bodied men given the continued unequal distribution of domestic labour between men and women.

In the formal sphere, in the statutory, voluntary and private sectors, women are key service providers, at least in the front line of service delivery (EOC, 1988). As is discussed in greater detail in, for example, Chapters 3, 7 and 8, much of the increase in women's labour market participation in the post-war years has been in relatively low-paid work in the social service sector – in health care, the personal social services and education, for example (Rein, 1985; Cousins, 1987). In Chapter 11 Brunsdon and May also point to the reliance of private welfare providers on the low-paid labour of women.

As users, paid social service workers and as unpaid care-givers, women are thus, as Fraser (1989: 147) notes, the principal subjects of social welfare in a 'feminised terrain'. Given their dominance in this terrain it might be expected that women should be in a position to frame and shape the services, in Hernes' third status as participants in political processes. However, this is not the case in the United King-dom. While women constitute the majority of the welfare workforce, vertical occupa-tional segregation within welfare services such as education, health care and the personal social services means that the agencies are managed principally by men, as Deem, Foster, Davis and Hooper suggest in this volume. In the more formal political

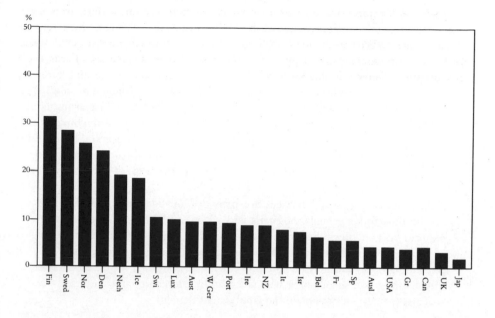

Figure 1.2 Women in national legislatures, 1983. (Source: Norris, 1986: 115)

arenas which shape and resource welfare policy, particularly in central and local government, the dominant players are men. As Hernes argues 'in the political process women are recipients and men are participants' (1987: 76). Figure 1.2 shows that women were under-represented in national legislatures in the 1980s. In the 1990s the United Kingdom's very low position remains almost unchanged. In the Civil Service, women and particularly women of minority ethnic origin, are concentrated in the lowest grades (EOC, 1988). Similar patterns of under-representation of women, especially Black women, are found in British local government, particularly in respect of key political positions such as chairs or convenors of committees. The position is summarised by Webster (1985: 91) as follows:

> Three key groups of actors within the local authority who are involved in policy-making processes – elected members, senior officials and union representatives – are all dominated by men. Clearly there may be people within these groups who are concerned about issues which affect women and instances where they fight to protect these interests. . . . However, the marked absence of women in formal positions of power in the policy-making arena means that there is a high probability that these interests will be poorly represented.

The position, then, is one in which women are poorly represented in formal, political and policy-making arenas, yet are key stakeholders in social policy as users and providers of services. The assumptions about women and their roles which are embodied in social policies, the terms on which welfare is delivered, the extent to which it meets their needs or extends choice and its consequences, intended and unintended, are all of central importance in the lives of many women and are explored in subsequent chapters in this volume.

2 'Race', gender and social policy

Shafquat Nasir

Introduction

The main purpose of this chapter is to provide a framework for understanding, exploring and analysing four major issues: the dominance within western feminist theory and practice of the views, norms, perspectives and political agendas of White[1] women, the inter-relationship/interaction of 'race'[2] and gender in relation to welfare needs, the ideological foundations of social policy and the welfare state as it operates in contemporary British society.

My aim in doing this is quite specifically and deliberately *not* to add statistical or factual information about Black women's experience of welfare as a discrete self-contained chapter in a book. Too often separate chapters on Black women are merely tokenistic – a way of avoiding the criticism of ignoring 'race' without questioning the marginalisation of 'race' at a theoretical level within the frameworks used in feminist analyses. Since all the contributors in this book have been asked to address differences in relation to 'race'/ethnicity, class, age, sexuality and disability, empirical material on the relative position of Black women in relation to major policy areas and issues can be found in specific chapters.[3] There are furthermore a number of studies both quantitative and qualitative from which such empirical material can be extracted.[4] While this chapter focuses mainly on theoretical questions and issues, references to research are given throughout to assist further study.

As issues related to racial/ethnic differences have traditionally been obscured and marginalised within both social policy analysis and feminist writing, the first task is to explore some of the reasons for this exclusion in each of these areas of study. Particular attention will be paid to the ways in which both theoretical and practical feminist projects in the west have assumed a universal female experience based on an implicit assumption that White women's experiences and issues are the norm.

In order to illustrate the way in which the experiences of Black women have been marginalised, some main themes and debates that have been explored by feminist writers on the British welfare state will be examined. The extent to which the position and experiences of Black women have been taken into account and how they are positioned in relation to the concerns and political agenda set out by feminist writers on social policy will be examined. This will be followed by consideration of the impact of social policies upon the lives of Black women, outlining the differences in their experience as compared with that of White women. The contribution to this debate of what has come to be called Black feminism will then be further examined since in constructing criteria for an analysis that does not assume race neutrality it is important that the problems of false universality, additionalism and notions of homogeneity are not repeated in discussions about the position of Black women. Black women in Britain have diverse histories, backgrounds and perceptions, which clearly have an impact on individual Black women's experience of social welfare. Consideration of differences between Black women is not only vital in attempts to draw an accurate picture of Black women in this country, but is also important at a theoretical level in formulating an analysis of the relative importance of other variables such as age, class, sexuality and disability.

Finally, some prerequisites are outlined for developing a clearer conceptual framework which is able to deal more flexibly with difference between women and within which specific pieces of factual information and research findings might be placed.

'Race' in the context of social policy analysis

There is a general tendency within the western intellectual/academic project of separating issues in order to study them, which has contributed to fragmentation in relation to concepts of social identity and the reification of unitary single-factor categories within discussions of social divisions (Anthias, 1990; Afshar and Maynard, 1994). This results in the construction of an 'either–or' dichotomy which not only means that an individual and, for the purposes of this chapter, a Black woman, is considered *either* as a woman *or* as a Black person,[5] but also limits the possibilities for exploring and understanding differences within these artificially constructed groups. As each group is treated as though it were discrete, self-contained and internally homogeneous, the possibility of an identity across groups is foreclosed (Rattansi, 1992; Brewer, 1993).

Within the discipline of social policy the problem is compounded by the history of idealism and empiricism in post-war writing and the late arrival of theoretical and materialist accounts in the 1970s, prior to which there was a strong tendency towards privileging facts and figures rather than the construction of explanatory theoretical frameworks. This is one reason why the recognition of feminist and anti-racist perspectives has been slow. However, development of the latter has been a great deal slower and there seems to be greater reluctance to include anti-racist or Black perspectives than there is to include material on women's disadvantage and feminist perspectives. Williams' book *Social Policy: A critical introduction* (1989) is unique in its in-depth consideration of 'race' and anti-racist perspectives within the discipline of social policy. Williams points out the following:

- There are clear links to be drawn between the demise of the British Empire and the concepts and principles underpinning the post-war welfare state and its narrow conception of citizenship.
- The major migrations of Black peoples to Britain in the 1950s and 1960s were often promoted by the needs of welfare agencies for cheap workers, yet the welfare needs of these workers were not considered or planned for.
- Entitlement and access to provision have been, and continue to be, heavily affected by 'race' and nationality.
- Black people experience welfare agencies differently from the White/indigenous population.
- Universalism within theories underpinning welfare often results in services being inappropriate to Black people.

There has been very little acknowledgement of this in mainstream social policy texts and journals. Hall suggests that this general phenomenon can in part be explained by 'an indigenous British racism in the post war period which begins with a profound historical forgetfulness . . . a kind of historical amnesia' (Hall, 1978: 25). The debate that occurred through the pages of the journal of *Critical Social Policy* during 1986 between Black and White members of the editorial collective and the work of people like Gurnah (1989) and Gordon (1986, 1989) illustrate clearly that within both the theory and the practice of welfare active marginalisation of 'race' and denial of the existence of racism are still a major problem.

The marginalisation of 'race' in western feminism and feminist critiques of welfare

Western feminism has based much of its argument for independent feminist analysis of the position of women in society on a critique of 'the masculinist truth-claim to universality or academic objectivity' (Spivak, 1986: 225). It has been argued that a false universalism has concealed the androcentric and masculinist perspectives within social, political and economic studies (Gunew, 1992; Walby, 1990b), Stanley (1991) and Smith (1988) have been among those who have shown how such biases have played a central role in the construction of research agendas and methodologies in the social sciences. Many feminists have therefore strongly objected to the practice of merely 'adding' women, their existence, interests and issues on to existing analyses and have argued that instead the epistemological bases of theoretical constructs need to be re-appraised, reworked and transformed in the light of feminist theory (Harding, 1987; Smith, 1988; Gunew, 1992).

Despite a spoken commitment to addressing women's inequality in society, however, in their concern to forge solidarity between women western feminists have largely failed to take into account both the existence and the position of Black women. Feminists have challenged dominant conceptions of women without giving due recognition to how, within western thinking, the term woman has been naturalised as the White woman of European descent. Thus the way in which dominant ideas are structured around this group's socio-cultural history, and the way in which Black women are not only perceived differently but also sometimes as opposite and other is not addressed (Carby, 1982; Parmar, 1988). Racialised gender stereotypes and their effects have very rarely been addressed by western feminists. This has resulted in a false universalism within feminist analysis itself (Amos and Parmar, 1984; Bhavnani, 1990; Aziz, 1992).

Feminists have often based their approach on assumptions and assertions that it is possible to separate experiences which are seen as specifically connected to gender inequality from other forces, that there is a substantial core within women that is almost unaffected by 'race', ethnicity and class. This has led to the criticism that feminist analyses also have a tendency towards reductionism and essentialism (Spelman, 1988; Gunew, 1992). What emerges from these theoretical tendencies is the naturalisation of the female subject, whose identity as woman is separated from other identities such as those based on 'race' and ethnicity. Since the liberal tradition within academia also obscures these two factors and feminists have not been able to divorce themselves from this paradigm, feminist analyses have displayed a strong tendency towards ethnocentrism and Eurocentrism (Bhavnani and Coulson, 1986; Spelman, 1988).

'Groups unequal in power are correspondingly unequal in their ability to make their standpoint known to both themselves and others' (Hill Collins, 1990: 26). Hill Collins makes an important point here about the production of knowledge which explains part of the reason why feminist theory has traditionally been marginalised, but also why the issues and concerns of a dominant group of women, White, middle and upper class, heterosexual and able-bodied, have shaped feminist thought in the western world and have predominated in feminist theory. Black women (and men), both historically and to a lesser extent currently, have not had equal access to the higher levels of education, far less than their White female counterparts, who in turn have had a great deal less access than White men (Zack-Williams and Dennis, 1994). Despite the evidence that there is increasing awareness of the role social identity plays in the construction of knowledge, change in the composition of the body of people engaged in academic enquiry and theory building has been and continues to be extremely slow. Theoretical frameworks that allow analysis of the interaction of 'race', gender, class and other factors have yet to be developed (Aziz, 1992).

The word 'feminist' refers directly only to one part of a person's identity – that based on sex and gender; her 'race', class, sexuality, age and ability are not covered by the term. Whilst some would argue that to be a feminist implicitly involves a commitment to liberation from all oppressive forces, the artificial separation of gendered identity and relations from other social constructs has led to a situation where the most optimistic outcome at the level of both theoretical frameworks and practice is in effect the mere addition of other identities involved in unequal power dynamics. Thus at the centre of feminist analysis is the 'pure', 'essential' woman. This has meant that the point at which the identity 'women' intersects/interacts with other variables is necessarily peripheral and thus the position of Black women is continuously marginalised 'so that when they are depicted it is as an exception' (Aziz, 1992: 297).

Many Black women have argued that Black and White women cannot adequately be subsumed within one unitary category and that the specificities of Black and White women's histories, geographical locations, socio-economic, cultural and political positions need to be far more rigorously documented and theorised before progress or transformation occurs within feminist/women's studies (Aziz, 1992; Brah, 1992; Bhavnani, 1994). Yet it is not enough to add Black women into existing frameworks and it is unhelpful to try to incorporate difference by merely extending and adding social categories to the labels given to different feminist positions, for example Black feminist, Black lesbian feminist, working-class Black lesbian feminist. Attempts to analyse the inter-relationship of these factors, which have each been fairly rigidly defined, often with an assumption of clear boundaries and internal homogeneity, have reflected this additionalism (Afshar and Maynard, 1994).

At first terms like 'double' then 'triple' oppression were used; more recent and sophisticated analyses refer to the way in which race, class and other factors reconstitute the way in which oppressions are manifest (Williams, 1989; Anthias and Yuval-Davis, 1992). Several authors even refer to multiple layers of identity and intersection of factors. However, the core concept of woman is rarely displaced from the centre of the discussion. Anthias and Yuval-Davis (1992) and Aziz (1992), for example, carefully examine the various formulas that are used, yet come to the conclusion that at both analytical and concrete levels interactions and inter-relationships are named rather than theorised.

Tensions within feminist theory in relation to 'race' are not only created by the existence and claims of Black women, but also Black men. An undifferentiated analysis of the category man and the notion of patriarchy are as problematic and perhaps a little more threatening to address, than the unitary category of woman (Johnson-Reagan, 1983; Bhavnani, 1994; Zack-Williams and Dennis, 1994). Feminism, in common with many other movements which are based on one part of social identity has at its heart a general and perhaps rather crude understanding of power which, if operationalised in analysis, can act as an interpretive framework that is rigid, totalising and teleological. Cohen goes as far as to claim that such approaches:

> explain the actions or attitudes of particular individuals or groups, and the
> meaning of particular events, as the expression of an over-determining social

totality – 'capital society', 'patriarchy', or 'the white power structure' – which supervenes in every case to determine the form of all social eventualities. (Cohen, 1992: 77)

Although a main concern of feminists has been aimed at making women visible in order to address the interests and issues pertaining to women, if the intention of feminism is to counter oppression this does not excuse the absence of consideration of the position of Black men. The disinclination to address power differences between men, and in particular power differences between women and men where women can be seen to be more powerful, is often based on the discomfort resulting from the position of women being displaced from its central position in the hierarchy of oppressions sometimes explicitly, but more often implicitly constructed in feminist analysis. Furthermore just as constructions of women's sexuality vary according to 'race' – so do those of men. Black men, particularly those of African descent, have been constructed as super-masculine, as rapists, as sexual aggressors and thus they are seen as embodying the worst aspects of maleness that feminists challenge (Wallace, 1979; Bhavnani, 1990). Yet an analysis of the position of Black men is vital to our understanding of both Black women's lives and political projects and indeed of the dynamics of power in our society, as Aziz notes:

Women oppressed and exploited by racism and/or imperialism have some interests in common with their menfolk – as opposed to white western men and women . . . this maps out a vast area of complex solidarities, contradictions and struggles which women, seen globally, inhabit. (Aziz, 1992: 291)

Feminist critiques of welfare and their inadequacy in accounting for and analysing the experiences of Black women

It has been mentioned earlier that Black women do not fit into dominant ideas about women's (naturalised as White) position within western advanced capitalist societies. Much has been written by feminists on patriarchal ideologies and attitudes relating to the roles of women, in particular their position in the family, their sexuality and reproduction. However, the construction of women as dependants of men and as gaining their value in society through motherhood have been based on the historical development of the rights and roles of White, often middle-class, British women (Williams, 1989). Non-European/non-White women have been positioned as 'other' to White women, their position being conceptualised in direct relation to how they differ from White women.

In an analysis of the relative position of White women compared to Black women of Asian and Afro-Caribbean descent the White woman occupies central ground on a continuum between submissive and aggressive. It is almost as though the Asian woman is made invisible and excluded from the dominant conception of 'woman' by virtue of not having an independent status as a human being in her own right, as she is seen to be ultimately submissive to, or an adjunct of, Asian men (Amos and Parmar, 1984; Parmar, 1988; Brah, 1992), whilst women of African descent, particularly those with a history of slavery, have lost their femininity because they are seen to be independent from men of their racial/cultural group, or even conceptualised as a threat to them, when they are seen as emasculating/castrating Black men (Wallace, 1979).

In order to gain an understanding of the way in which Black women's identity has been constructed it is necessary to delineate the development and perpetuation of racist ideologies in the western world. Davis (1982), for instance, argued that Black women are anomalies within the ideology of femininity that was developed in the nineteenth century. The picture of women as 'nurturing mothers, gentle companions and housekeepers for their husbands' (p. 5) was entirely incompatible with the view of Black women, whose whole reason for being was to work; they may have been nurturing nannies, ladies companions and house-servants to White families, but they were 'only incidentally a wife and mother' to their own family (p. 5). Though Davis is referring to slavery in America the impact of racist ideology did not stop when Black people won their freedom, nor was the ideology contained within the American continent.

In Britain, Black women are often seen as immigrant workers (or wives of immigrant workers). Again they are seen primarily as a unit of labour and, as Carby (1982: 215) comments, the ideology of Black women as servants is as strong as that of women as carers. Furthermore, Bruegel (1989), Mama (1984), Hallett (1989), Cook and Watt (1992) and Phizacklea (1994) show that in terms of their position in the labour market Black women are affected by complex divisions that can be described as vertical and horizontal workforce segregation affected by gender-, 'race-' and class-based factors. These do not result in a simple adding of factors but interlock with notions of femininity and family, so that Black women are more likely to work full-time as opposed to their White counterparts, who are predominantly found in part-time work. The latter are expected to work around the caring needs of their families while the former, as Carby puts it, are 'seen to fail as mothers precisely because of their position as workers' (1982: 219). They are, therefore, denied any of the 'positive' status or treatment which results from the orientation in British social policy to familism (Williams, 1989).

Black women's needs have not been addressed either specifically in relation to their position as workers with childcare needs or more generally within social policy. This is likely to be a result, at least in part, of the assumptions that firstly Black people should not be dependent on the state, as they are often not seen as full citizens (Gordon and Newnham, 1985; Gilroy 1987; Gordon, 1989), and secondly of racist ideologies pertaining to each group. It is expected that African–Caribbean women should be self-sufficient, whilst Asian women should be wholly dependent on their husbands, their extended family and close-knit community (Parmar, 1988; Brah, 1994). Paradoxically, Black women are also seen as scroungers on state welfare. The comparatively higher proportion of African–Caribbean women who are single parents is exaggerated and stereotyped through media representations and in public opinion. Asian women, on the other hand, are said to 'breed like rabbits', having children in order to gain access to welfare funds. Thus the contradictory tensions involved in racist ideology are clear. Black women's higher participation in full-time work compared to White women is interpreted as Black people taking the jobs of White people, yet they are also seen as swelling the dole queues and being lazy and unproductive at the same time as producing too many children, for whom they expect the state to take responsibility.

Beyond issues related to access to resources, Black women's qualitative experience of welfare is also different from that of White women. Black women have been reported to be more likely to be given long-term contraception, abortions and sterilisations (Bryan *et al.*, 1985; Williams, 1989). This is partly due to Black people's presence being unwanted in this country and partly because women of African descent are seen as promiscuous and Asian women are seen as having high fertility without adequate consideration of contraception or family planning.

There also seems to be a pattern of under-research and lack of knowledge amongst medical personnel about conditions more commonly suffered by Black people, the incidence of sickle-cell anaemia in those of African descent, for example (Grimsley and Bhat, 1988). Also the family-planning side of health care in conditions such as sickle-cell anaemia are more heavily emphasised than those related to prevention and treatment of sickle-cell crisis, which supports the suggestion that there is a preoccupation with using welfare to control the Black population rather than to genuinely address health needs (Manchester Law Centre Immigration Handbook No. 6, 1987).

These views of Black women are connected to and exacerbated by what has been named both in America and this country as 'Black cultural pathology' and 'Black family pathology' (Lawrence, 1982). As Black people with different cultural backgrounds have different types of stereotypes applied to them this will be explored in greater detail in the section on differences among Black women. However, it is possible to identify some common characteristics involved in this pathologisation.

Black cultural pathology refers to a process by which structural inequalities and the effect of past inequalities are ignored and the explanation for the statistically higher frequency of Black people in poverty, inadequate housing, poor health status, educational underachievement and for some groups higher rates of social work intervention, rests on notions that Black people have dysfunctional families and cultures which produce and reproduce such poor welfare conditions. Black women who are mothers are seen as central to this reproduction of culture through their child-rearing. The details of how this is applied to different cultural groups will be explored later; however, the most important point is that *all* are seen as deviant and inferior to white family norms.

It is important to examine the way in which Black cultural pathologies serve to reduce the emphasis on racism and divide Black people as an analytical category and as a political pressure group (Rattansi, 1992). When one group suffers a particular type of discrimination and another does not this can be used to counter the claim of racism; so for instance Black children of African–Caribbean origin are said to have little motivation in relation to their schooling, to have more disruptive behaviour and to be less able academically. Asian children are seen as highly motivated, hard-working (though not always successful) and deferential. Thus it can be claimed that the problem is not racism, as both groups of Black children are not affected equally; the fault must therefore lie with the African–Caribbean family and culture. This is, however, a false dichotomy. If one were to study the educational achievement of Asian children in Bradford, the majority of whom come from families originating in rural working-class areas of Pakistan, the situation regarding the educational position of Asian children is far less optimistic. Moreover, alongside notions of the higher motivation of Asian students there are also assumptions about their ability to communicate in English, and, for girls, the alleged restrictive practices of their overprotective parents are thought to have a negative impact on their learning environment and experience of schooling (Parmar, 1988).

A prerequisite of cultural pathology is the belief in homogeneity within communities – whereby a whole group can be seen as sharing similar characteristics, views and needs. Therefore when consultation by welfare agencies and policy makers does take place with 'minority groups' issues around representation are rarely addressed. The needs of a few individuals, often men and often in a higher class position, are the ones that are articulated and communicated to policy makers. Not only are different cultural ethnic groups in a position of competing for resources, but also the diversity within these groups makes competition more intense – expressed needs are subject to claims and counter-claims. Whilst it is clearly important that the different needs of different groups are recognised, the level and intensity of the competition mean that individual claims become the priority of groups and policy makers. The danger in this is that questions related to the fact that mainstream services do not meet the needs of particular groups, or that these groups share a common position of marginalisation and disadvantage are not addressed (Cain and Yuval-Davis, 1990).

Western feminists have tended not to look at these specific ways in which Black women's experience of welfare differs from their own, the way in which, as Bhavnani and Coulson (1986) put it, the 'state deals differently with different women'. This has led to a one-dimensional and therefore oversimplified feminist analysis of welfare. Yet feminists have not only excluded such factors from their macro-analysis but also, on the occasions when they have addressed the needs of Black women, added to notions of Black women as problems and victims (Carby, 1982; James and Busia, 1993). Attitudes of feminist activists are also prone to this tendency, for instance the responses to arranged marriages which depict Asian women as helpless and passive (Parmar, 1982; Mama, 1989). Black women are too often depicted in feminist theory as 'the exception, the special case, the puzzle, more oppressed or exotic anomaly' (Aziz, 1992: 297). Their strengths and struggles are rarely recognised, either in terms of their ability to manage and survive the many forces which work against them, or as parts of communities resisting racism (Williams, 1989).

Feminists have argued that the 'welfare state reinforces a particular view of femininity and a particular type of family, not just in its detailed practices but also in the ideas it generates' (Pascall, 1983: 6). This is certainly the case, yet White feminists writing on welfare have also reinforced particular views and norms; by using a white perspective and universalising it they have sometimes pathologised Black women and their families, seeing them either as victims or as problems. More often, however, they have completely excluded Black women from their frame of reference. (The following books, which together constitute the bulk of textbooks on women and welfare, contain little or no reference to 'Black women', 'ethnic minority women' or 'racism': Wilson (1977) *Women and the Welfare State*; Ungerson (1985) *Women and Social Policy: A reader*; Dale and Foster (1986) *Feminists and State Welfare*; Pascall (1986) *Social Policy: A feminist analysis*; Dalley (1988) *Ideologies of Caring: Rethinking community and collectivism*; Maclean and Groves (1991) *Women's Issues in Social Policy*.) On the whole, then, feminist critiques of welfare have neither represented nor addressed the needs of Black women.

'Black feminism'

The majority of those who have questioned the false universalism of western feminism and have been critical of its inability to deal adequately with issues around 'race' have been Black women, some of whom have referred to themselves as 'Black feminists'. This new identity category has now begun to be outlined in some texts on feminism/feminisms.[6] Some of the main issues raised within this category are briefly outlined below:

- Refusal to accept oppositional dichotomies involving either/or formulations in relation to understanding 'race', gender and class dynamics.
- At a theoretical level suggesting that the central fixed position of patriarchy and the use of a universal category man are problematic. Firstly, this is because it assumes all men have power over all women. The differences between the power of White men and Black men are significant, and in some ways at least White women have more power than Black men. Secondly, the disinclination to analyse differences between women because they are conceptualised as a unitary category means that White feminists have not addressed their own power, its use and abuse.
- Challenging essentialism, reductionism, ethnocentrism and Eurocentrism in feminist theory and practice outlining the way in which these tendencies make Black women's lives either invisible or a deviation from the norm. These factors along with the reluctance to deal with issues of race constitute racism through exclusion, marginalisation and distortion of Black women's realities. This also clearly undermines the claim that a major objective of feminism is the liberation of all women.
- Because race has been undertheorised by White feminists they have not challenged racist thinking and are therefore in danger of uncritically accepting dominant

ideologies in relation to Black women. This then leads to the description and analysis of pathology.

There are differences between the authors who have contributed to these critiques, particularly in terms of their allegiance to feminism and how they conceptualise 'race' in relation to gender and class (see Williams, 1989, and for general differences in analyses of race and class Anthias, 1990; Anthias and Yuval-Davis, 1992; James and Busia, 1993). While these critiques can enhance feminist analysis or challenge them at a fundamental level, they have also had 'a central role in the development of a post-modern critique of the self' (Aziz, 1992: 304).

There are, however, some problems that can arise from Black feminism itself adopting a fixed position beyond the critique of exclusionary tendencies within west-ern feminism. It may be, for instance, that differences between Black women are not emphasised, understood or analysed. There seem to be a number of reasons for this, the first of which is the time at which many of these critiques were written. Throughout the 1980s critiques of multiculturalism became popular amongst aca-demics and activists, since multiculturalism had an emphasis on difference without an analysis of power. The fact of racism and the assumption of White superiority that led all cultures other than British/European to be seen as inferior were obscured. It was felt that politically it was important for Black people to unite, to make connections across cultural and ethnic groupings. Whilst this common front is a necessary compo-nent of resistance, more recent work on 'race' has suggested that this reduces Black peoples lives to victimhood, subjects of analysis within the frame of reference con-structed by traditional western thinking (Rattansi, 1992; P. Gilroy, 1993).

Secondly, for Black/anti-racist academics the task of correcting biases within their disciplines was a massive one, with few people able and willing to take it on. So, whilst there were at least limited opportunities to explore and to write about the marginalisation of race and racism within particular subjects it had to be contained in singular chapters in books and the odd article in journals; the pressure is always to try and do everything, rarely has there been the room to proceed from resistance/critique to building a sense of 'radical black subjectivity', which hooks discusses in *Yearning* (1990; see also Hill Collins, 1990).

This is now a very important project if false universalism, essentialism and notions of communities internally homogeneous with clear fixed boundaries are to be avoided in analyses of Black people. As Aziz argues:

> What needs to be placed at the heart of discourse on 'race' is a history which allows Black people the complexity, passion, intelligence and contradictions of thought, action and word that white people are implicitly [and automatically] credited with when Black people are seen as victims or problems. (1992: 295)

The questioning of the notion of an essential Black subject can also assist the develop-ment of clearer definitions and avoid the exclusion of certain groups (Madood, 1988; Anthias and Yuval-Davis, 1992; Brah, 1992).

Differences among Black women: implications for social policy analysis

The largest groups of Black women in Britain come from three different continents, within which there are major regional differences; they come from different class backgrounds and have a wide variety of religious and cultural beliefs. Furthermore they have different historical links to Britain through slavery and colonialism, and have had different migration patterns. Clearly, these factors have an impact on Black women's relative positions and experiences in relation to economic, political and social structures and dominant ideologies in Britain, to their welfare needs and policy responses to such needs.

The social construction and control of women's sexuality have been a central concern for feminists. It is seen as particularly important in relation to the formulation of the claim that 'the personal is the political' so strongly articulated in twentieth-century feminism. However, the vast majority of feminist writing on sexuality has assumed a universal, unitary category of woman – perhaps it is the clearest example of the tendency within feminism towards essentialism and reductionism as the female body is the focus of analysis. Yet Black women's sexuality has been constructed very differently, even oppositionally to that of White women. One way to conceptualise this is by use of a continuum on which White women occupy the central ground between sexually submissive and sexually aggressive, with women of Asian descent being most often placed within the category of sexually submissive and women of African descent being characterised as sexually aggressive (Thomas and Sillen, 1976; Marshall, 1994).

Therefore sexuality can be seen as central not only to women's oppression but also to the construction of racist ideologies, forming one of the most fundamental reference points of the identity of the 'other', both in the past (H. Bhaba in Fanon, 1986; Gilman, 1992) and currently within popular culture (P. Gilroy, 1993). Furthermore, it is possible to trace direct links between such notions and the construction and implementation of social policies: for instance Thomas and Sillen show how 'a preoccupation with sexual themes haunts both the popular and professional literature' (1976: 101) in American psychiatry.

Table 2.1 outlines the different ways in which the sexuality of Black women of African and Asian descent has been conceptualised, showing how such ideas impact upon social policies. Clearly, welfare professionals do not operate within a social vacuum, they are influenced by dominant ideologies and media representations. In social work, for instance, Dominelli (1986) states that norms related to the White middle-class family are the standard by which others are judged. Table 2.2 outlines the way in which actual differences and popular assumptions in relation to Black families impact upon social policy and the practices of welfare professionals.

Table 2.1 Differences in the construction of Black women's sexuality

	Women of African origin	Women of Asian origin
Historical foundations for dominant western constructions of Black women's sexuality	The rape of female slaves was justified in terms of (i) the need to control them, (ii) their sexual insatiability and inherent promiscuity. Early studies of African women by orientalists and anthropologists placed a heavy emphasis on their sexuality, for example the exaggerated depictions of Hottentot females (Gilman, 1992).	Sometimes characterised as exotic sexual creatures by orientalists; however, such views do not seem to be commonly accepted or to have influenced current ideas about the Asian women who settled in this country after the Second World War. Asian women are more often portrayed as non-sexual or sexually passive and submissive to Asian men. In discussions around sexuality Asian women are invisible.
Current dominant notions	Women of African descent are still thought of as more sexual and more promiscuous than White women.	Asian women are still seen as passive. There are very few images of Asian women as sexual beings. They are not seen as sexually active or assertive and therefore are not thought to make sexual choices such as lesbianism.
Impact on construction of social policies and experience of implementation	Greater control of reproduction through more frequent use of long-term contraceptives, abortions and sterilisations. Increased emphasis on social work intervention for young women in care. The mind/body split also manifests itself in the field of education, where girls of African descent are seen as unacademic but good at sports.	Greater control of reproduction but based on notions around fertility and lack of concern/control re family planning. The virginity tests carried out by the Home Office to establish the primary purpose of marriage when Asian women have tried to enter the country to join prospective husbands are clearly based on the idea that Asian women are not sexually active outside marriage. Evidence that information about AIDS and HIV are not getting through to certain groups of Asian women may also be influenced by this.

Table 2.2 The impact of common-sense notions of Black women/families on the implementation of social policies

	Women of African origin	Women of Asian origin
Actual differences	Higher percentage of one-parent and female-headed households than both British people and Asian people. Higher rates of participation in full-time work, and working longer hours and more likely to work unsociable hours.	Lower percentage of one-parent and female-headed households. Higher rates of participation in full-time work and working longer hours. Higher participation in homeworking.
Common-sense notions	The number of one-parent families is often exaggerated, as are discipline-related problems said to be due to the lack of a stable family background and the absence of a father figure. Because structural inequalities resulting in the necessity to work more hours (at a lower rate of pay than the average for White women) are often not given due consideration, the efforts of African–Caribbean women to juggle the demands of full-time, often heavy-duty work with raising a family are ignored. Instead they are pathologised and said to be neglectful in relation to their parental responsibilities.	The Asian family is seen as close-knit, self-sufficient, insular and introspective – strong to the extent of being repressive Asian females are seen as subservient first to their father and then to their husband. The rate of Asian women's economic participation does not fit well in this framework and is often ignored. The attitude towards Asian women is often patronising. In terms of their relationships with their families they are seen as being without power, and are sometimes accused of not being able to influence or supervise their children adequately because of this.
Impact on social policy	There are a disproportionate number of African–Caribbean children in care. The children also have greater contact with the police, and there is evidence that they are dealt with more severely if they come into contact with any part of the criminal justice system. Stereotypes about disruptive behaviour affect teachers' perceptions and responses to Black African–Caribbean children. This in turn affects expectations and actual academic performance. However, the parents of the children are often held wholly responsible for their children's underachievement and negative attitude towards education. The combination of stereotypes about African–Caribbean women's sexuality and their supposed lack of interest in their children's welfare or lack of parenting skills justifies social work intervention and policies like those that operate in some states in the United States, where Black women's access to welfare is made conditional to them having long-term contraceptives implanted.	The notion that the Asian community is self-sufficient and insular has been used to excuse lack of service provision, as it is assumed that they would rather provide for themselves. There is relatively little social work intervention. Teachers complain that children from poorer Asian families where access of the mother to English language is limited are inadequately prepared for school. There is also a claim that Asian parents have unrealistically high expectations of their children that are damaging through the pressure they create. It is the way in which the Asian woman is depicted as a victim of arranged marriages that wins support for the Home Office intervening in intimate affairs such as those involved in the establishment of the primary purpose of marriage.

Developing theoretical frameworks linking 'race', gender and other variables

Clearly the use of a concept of woman as a universal, unitary category in attempts to understand and analyse the relationship between women and the welfare state is problematic. White women/western feminists need to recognise themselves within their analyses as 'raced' people, if they are truly concerned about decreasing the invisibility of Black women in their work. Currently Black women are being positioned as subjects of study, if their needs and perspectives are acknowledged at all. The discrete chapters that exist within a very small number of books on women and social policy are merely 'added' into the texts; they leave the theoretical framework of a reductionist, essentialist and Eurocentric western feminism intact.

Differences among women, and indeed differences between particular groups of women, such as Black women, need to be not only acknowledged but allowed to challenge and transform the existing theoretical bases upon which feminist analyses of the state and welfare are built.

When issues of difference are discussed within feminist texts, the debate is often preceded or followed by questions about whether any statements/claims on group identity can be made. Is there not, as Brah (1992: 126) suggests: 'a danger that the specificity of a particular experience may itself become an expression of essentialism?' In order to progress from this point Brah makes a distinction between 'social relations at the level of the social structure', an analysis of which is crucial 'when addressing the structural, political, and historical basis of the commonality of experience', and experience based 'primarily in terms of collective histories' (p. 141) and biographies. These two levels are often conflated, and therefore attempts to deal with difference are prematurely halted as a very limited, deterministic and rigid set of theories about structural inequalities are forced to be the explanatory base for extremely diverse and complex ideas, perceptions and experiences. Whilst a distinction needs to be made between the two, which is crucial to any project in which an understanding of difference and overdeterministic models are to be avoided, 'in practice, the everyday of lived experience and experience as a social relation do not exist in mutually exclusive spaces' (Brah, 1992: 141).

Within analyses of social inequalities in the field of social policy, particularly when gender, 'race' and other variables are included as specific dimensions of such inequalities, insights into identity, ideology and culture are needed. Furthermore, in order to move beyond cataloguing discrete manifestations of discrimination, describing policies and outlining political perspectives it is necessary to integrate an awareness of: 'the significance of complex interpretive *frameworks* through which events, processes and facts are *constructed*. Experience, that is, is produced, rather than simply registered' (Rattansi, 1992: 33). This not only enables a number of important factors to be included in analysis, but also, as Aziz notes: 'Such a perspective can save identity from "mummifying" by challenging us self-consciously to deconstruct our identities. This act of deconstruction is political, as it exposes the intricate operations of power that constitute subjectivity' (1992: 304).

Acknowledgements

I would like to thank Susannah Wells, Kate McGowan and Caroline Ukoumunne for their support and for their comments on the subject and content of this chapter.

Notes

1. Capital letters are used when talking about White/Black people as the terms refer to social-political identities rather than being purely descriptive terms (see also Williams, 1989: ix–x).
2. The term 'race' has been placed in inverted commas as it is a social construction rather than a biological/genetic/physical category (see also Williams, 1989: ix–x; Donald and Rattansi, 1992: 1).
3. There are two reasons why these differences have not been explored in this chapter: firstly, given the restrictions on space, only one difference could be explored in any depth; and secondly, theoretical work on the way these factors inter-relate needs to be developed further before it can be integrated successfully into a chapter of this nature.
4. There are of course methodological problems with research into 'race'. Some of the issues related to this are discussed in Bhat *et al.* (1988); issues specifically related to research about Black women are addressed by Bhavnani (1994), Akeroyd (1994), Mama (1989) and Ladner (1971).
5. This is a position neatly summarised by Hull *et al.* (1981) in the title of their book, *All the Women Are White, All the Blacks Are Men – but Some of Us Are Brave.*
6. Challenges to the unitary category of woman used in feminist analysis and the influence of postmodern writing on difference have caused a number of those involved with feminism to talk of a number of feminist positions and approaches – this is one attempt to deal with difference between women – for instance, Humm (1993) *Feminisms: A reader.*

3   *Women and employment*

Claire Callender

Introduction

Just as the study of social policy, until recently, ignored the importance of gender so, too, has it often overlooked labour market issues and employment policies, in particular. This is due, in part, to its preoccupation with the provision of certain services supplied directly or indirectly through the state and, in part, to the narrow way in which social policy has been conceptualised. Yet employment remains the main route out of poverty and dependency on the state – it is vital in avoiding poverty and disadvantage.

Issues about employment rest more easily with economists whose perspectives dominate than with social policy analysts. Now more than ever, however, the boundaries between social and employment policies are blurring: for instance, today employment and the receipt of social security benefits are not mutually exclusive, but they were when the focus of concern was the lack of income from employment. How do we classify training policies? Are they social or economic policies or both?

The purpose of this chapter is to explore recent government employment policies and their impact on women. The first part examines women's changing position in the labour market and highlights the implications for policy development. The second considers the barriers women face in access to employment and in obtaining better jobs. This includes an assessment of policies aimed at improving women's

Table 3.1 Women and men in the labour force: 1971–2001

	Women		Men	
	Number (000)	%	Number (000)	%
1971	9,332	37.5	15,563	62.3
1981	10,598	40.4	15,644	59.6
1991	12,191	43.4	15,886	56.6
1993	12,215	43.8	15,645	56.2
2001	13,074	45.1	15,880	54.6

Source: Employment Department (1993a)

access. The third section considers the limitations of the model of social policy underpinning the analysis which assumes that social policies alone can substantially eradicate the problems women encounter in the labour market.

Women's position in the labour market

How many women are in the labour force?

The number of women in the labour force has been increasing since the 1950s and this trend will continue into the next century. There are currently over 12.2 million women in the labour force, a figure which is expected to rise to 13 million in 2001 (Table 3.1). By contrast, the number of men in the labour force (currently 15.7 million) has been declining. As a result, women now account for 44 per cent of the labour force and their share is projected to increase to 45 per cent by the end of the decade.

These trends have implications for employment policies. Between now and the end of the century more than three out of four people who enter the labour market will be women. Unless their needs are taken into account it is difficult to see how the economy's requirement for skilled labour can be met. Moreover, most of the jobs growth over the next two decades will be in highly skilled, professional and managerial jobs: jobs where women are currently under-represented. So to meet future employment needs and to effectively match the demand for certain types of jobs with the labour supply, changes will be required to get women into these occupations in sufficient numbers to meet demand.

What proportion of women of working age are working?

The trends outlined above reflect enduring and continuing changes in the pattern of women's labour force participation. More than 71 per cent of women of working age

(16–59 years) in Britain are currently economically active compared with 64 per cent in 1981 and 43 per cent in 1951 (Hakim, 1993). By contrast, men's current economic activity rate of 86 per cent has dropped from a high of 96 per cent in 1951 (Employment Department, 1992b; Sly, 1993). By 2001 women's economic activity rate is projected to rise to 74 per cent while for men it is projected to decline to 84 per cent. Thus there is increasing convergence in the pattern of labour force participation of men and women, even if their overall experience of the labour market remains very different.

Which women work?

Age

There are considerable differences in the economic activity rates of women depending upon their age.[1] These differences are related to the stage women are in their life cycle and, in particular, the presence of children. Recent changes in the age composition of the female workforce reflect the overall growth in women working, especially those aged 25–44. In 1981, 57 per cent of women aged 25–34 and 68 per cent of those aged 35–44 were economically active. This has now risen to 69 per cent and 77 per cent respectively. Moreover, it is precisely these age groups where the greatest projected increases are likely to occur (Employment Department, 1993a).

Dependent children

The expansion of women's employment can be attributed to the transformation in the labour force participation of women with young children (along with the increases in demand for certain types of labour). Marital status used to be the most important indicator of women's economic activity but this is no longer the case. Today responsibility for dependent children (i.e. under 16 years) is the most significant determinant of whether or not women work. In particular, the age of their youngest dependent child has a strong influence.

In 1993 the economic activity rate for women of working age with children was 63 per cent compared with 77 per cent for those without children. The activity rate was lowest for those with pre-school children and highest for those whose with school-age children (Table 3.2). Over the last decade, the proportion of women with no dependent children who were economically active rose from 74 to 77 per cent. For women with dependent children it was more marked (from 55 per cent to 63 per cent). For women with children age 0–4 years, however, the rise was even more substantial, from 37 per cent to 51 per cent (Table 3.2). If these trends continue, women will account for an increasing share of the labour force over the next decade and a high proportion of these women will be mothers of young children.

Table 3.2 Women's economic activity rates (percentage) by age of youngest dependent child and family type: 1984–93

	1984	1987	1990	1993
Women without dependent children	74	76	78	77
Lone mothers Child's age (years)				
0–4	28	30	31	30
5–10	60	57	58	54
11–15	68	67	68	73
Married mothers Child's age (years)				
0–4	39	44	52	55
5–10	66	70	74	75
11–15	75	77	79	81
All mothers Child's age (years)				
0–4	37	43	48	51
5–10	65	68	72	71
11–15	74	75	78	79
All women	66	69	71	71

Source: Labour Force Survey, Spring 1993

Lone parents

The one major exception of this growth of working mothers is amongst 1.2 million lone mothers, who represent 15 per cent of all mothers. Only 38 per cent of all lone parents were working in 1993 compared to 63 per cent of married mothers. Indeed their economic activity rates have actually fallen, unlike married mothers (Table 3.2). The proportion working dropped during the 1980s from 45 per cent in 1981 to 39 per cent in 1990 in contrast to married women where the proportions rose from 47 per cent to 60 per cent (Bartholomew *et al.*, 1992).

Lone parents today evidently face greater difficulties in entering the labour market than do married women. Their declining economic activity is associated with their increasing reliance on income support which, in part, is a reflection of the changing characteristics of lone parents. Lone parents on income support today are more likely than those in 1980 to be single, to be younger, to have pre-school-aged children, not to receive maintenance and to be living alone. Lone parents with these characteristics are more likely to claim benefit. Their characteristics, however, do not explain entirely the increase in their propensity to claim income support.

The proportion of lone parents in receipt of income support increased sharply in the early 1980s and the recession of the early 1990s.[2] This suggests that employment opportunities are important in determining the proportion of lone parents in receipt of benefit. Unlike other groups, however, lone parents failed to benefit from the economic boom of the late 1980s. It is unlikely, therefore, that employment growth, by itself, will be sufficient to ensure that lone parents enter the labour market in large numbers. They seem to face particular barriers to employment such as poor qualifications, lack of work experience and lack of affordable childcare.[3]

Women from ethnic minorities

Differences in the economic activity rates of ethnic majority and minority women appear quite marked, with 72 per cent of White women but only 54 per cent of ethnic minority women in the labour market.[4] There are important differences in the economic activity rates between ethnic minority communities (Table 3.3) and also within age groups for ethnic minority women (Jones, 1993). This reflects a mix of factors, including differences in the degree to which ethnic minority women have been born and brought up in Great Britain.

The biggest single difference in economic activity is that women from ethnic minorities tend not to undertake part-time work (see below). In 1991, 39 per cent of White women worked part-time compared with 26 per cent of ethnic minority women (Employment Department, 1993b). The Black female labour force is far more polarised between those not in paid employment and those working full-time. This difference cannot be explained by differences in childcare responsibilities (Bruegel, 1994). This suggests that they too face particular barriers to employment, including enduring discrimination and issues associated with their history of settlement and entry into jobs in labour-intensive industries in city areas which have been heavily affected by industrial restructuring and decline. Thus their economic activity rates have been affected by a combination of regional factors along with industrial/sector effects.

What are women's employment patterns?

Although men's and women's participation rates have been converging, there remain marked differences in their employment patterns. Most women still leave the labour

Table 3.3 Economic activity rates of women and men from ethnic minorities

Ethnic origin	Women		Men	
	Economically active		Economically active	
	Number (000)	%	Number (000)	%
White	15,325	72	16,796	86
Black	268	66	265	80
Indian	305	61	316	81
Pakistani/Bangladeshi	214	25	203	72
Mixed/other origins	202	58	209	76
All ethnic minorities	989	54	992	78

Source: Labour Force Survey, Spring 1993

market and their full-time jobs to have children and then return to part-time jobs. The amount of time, however, they take out of the labour market for child-bearing and child-rearing has changed dramatically in recent years. Between 1979 and 1988 the proportion of women returning to the labour force within nine months of the birth of their child increased from less than 40 per cent to 65 per cent (McRae, 1991).

Nevertheless, childbirth is still associated with downward occupational mobility especially amongst those who return to work part-time. So the jobs women acquire on re-entering the labour market often are at lower skill (and pay) levels than the jobs they occupied previously as full-time workers (Dex, 1987).

Women returners

There are no statistics specifically on women returners. The Labour Force Survey for 1992, however, demonstrates that two-thirds of women (3.28 million) who were economically inactive gave domestic commitments including looking after the family as the main reason for their inactivity. A year later, just under a fifth of these women had returned to the labour market. About two-thirds of these returners were aged between 25 and 39 years and had a child aged 0–4 years (compared to 39 per cent and 35 per cent respectively of all economically active women). On their return, around two-thirds found a job, most of which (82 per cent) were part-time. A third of the returners, however, were unemployed (Labour Force Survey, 1992/3, unpublished data).

Thus a major problem facing women returners is unemployment. These women are likely to face similar problems to unemployed women generally. However, they may face additional difficulties. For example, as a result of being outside the labour market for some time, their skills and qualifications may be outdated, they may lack confidence in themselves and their working environment. As importantly, by being confined primarily to the home, they may have lost contact with the social networks which are often vital for gaining a job (Callender, 1987).

Even where women returners do not face unemployment, they are likely to be distinct from other new entrants into the labour market and have different requirements: for example, they are likely to be older; to possess skills already, even if they need updating; and to have gained a wealth of experience while engaged in unpaid work in the home. These have to be acknowledged by the government and employers alike in their employment policies. The proportion of women returners is likely to continue to increase throughout the 1990s as more women spend less time out of the labour market. Some of the re-entry problems they face may decline if they spend less time away from paid employment and especially if they return to their previous employer (Hirsh *et al.*, 1992).

What is the composition of the female workforce

The female workforce is composed of employees, the self-employed and those on government schemes. A breakdown of their composition is provided in Table 3.4. It shows some dramatic differences between men and women.

Table 3.4 Composition of the female and male workforce: 1993

	Women		Men		Women as a % of those in the group
	Number (000)	%	Number (000)	%	%
Employees – full-time	5,488	47.5	10,316	67.7	34.7
Employees – part-time	4,260	36.9	564	3.7	88.3
Self-employed	718	6.2	2,210	14.5	24.5
Government schemes	115	1.0	222	1.5	34.1
Unpaid family workers	92	0.8	30	0.2	76.0
Unemployed (ILO)	879	7.6	1,892	12.4	31.7
Total	11,552	100.0	15,236	100.0	43.1

Source: Sly (1993) and author's calculations

Part-time workers

The overwhelming majority of women (84 per cent) are employees and of these over two-fifths work part-time. It is this high incidence of part-time work that distinguishes the female and male labour forces, since less than 5 per cent of men work part-time.

There has been a steady rise in the number of women working part-time since the 1950s. In 1951 only 11 per cent of women worked part-time and this jumped to 25 per cent in 1961 and 38 per cent a decade later (Hakim, 1993). By 1993, 44 per cent of all employed women worked part-time, representing 29 per cent of all women of working age compared with only 4 per cent of men. The problem with part-time work is that it often attracts poor conditions of employment, is excluded from certain employment rights and usually is low–paid and low-status work with limited opportunities for training and promotion.

Although there has been a consistent increase in the number of women working part-time, this has not been the case for full-time women workers. Part-time employment has fluctuated less than full-time employment. Indeed, the rise in women's economic activity, described at the beginning of this section, can be attributed to the expansion of women's part-time employment. As Hakim has commented:

> The much trumpeted rise in women's employment in Britain consisted entirely of the *substitution of part-time for full time jobs* from 1951 to the late 1980s . . . a genuine increase in women's full time work rates only occurred in the late 1980s, an increase that was temporarily halted by the recession of 1991/92. (Hakim, 1993: 102; italics in the original)

This trend in part-time employment is associated with the increasing propensity of women with children and other domestic commitments to take paid work. In 1993, 61 per cent of women with dependent children worked part-time compared with 32 per

Claire Callender

cent of those without children (Sly, 1993). Moreover, the trend is projected to continue. Indeed, future growth in female employment will almost wholly be accounted for by the expansion of part-time employment (Wilson, 1994).

The unemployed

The official monthly unemployment statistics for May 1994, based upon those claiming social security benefits, suggest that 13 per cent of men and 5 per cent of women were unemployed (Employment Department, 1994). Particularly at risk are women under the age of 25 and women from ethnic minorities. However, these figures underestimate the number of unemployed women and those experiencing long-term unemployment: they are biased and incomplete.

It has been estimated that one in four women who lose their jobs do not appear in the monthly claimant count. The Labour Force Survey (1993/4), which enumerates women who would like a job and are available for work,[5] includes almost two and a half times as many women as the claimant count. It puts the figure of female unemployment just under 1 million higher than the claimant count. It shows that 41 per cent of the unemployed are women whereas the monthly count suggests they form only 23 per cent.

This undercounting of unemployed women is especially important in terms of social and employment policies (Callender, 1992). Non-working women do not comply with our male-dominated conceptual framework for defining who is unemployed. If a man is healthy, of working age and not working, then he is unemployed. Women in a similar position, however, are not necessarily ascribed that status and so may be omitted from some statistics. A consequence is that women's experiences of unemployment are rendered invisible or marginalised and not considered a problem or worthy of comprehensive policy responses, unlike men's unemployment.

A practical manifestation of this exclusion is that women are under-represented on government training schemes, making up only a third of all participants (Table 3.4). As important, reliance on the official monthly statistics leads to an underestimation of the number of women who would like paid employment or access to government schemes.

Where do women work and what types of jobs do they have?

Another feature distinguishing women from men in the labour market is their different work and jobs. The great majority (83 per cent) of women work in service industries, compared with 56 per cent of men. Women with children and those who work part-time are even more concentrated in the services. Only 13 per cent of all working women and 8 per cent of part-timers work in manufacturing, compared with 28 per cent of men (Sly, 1993).

The segregation of men and women into different occupational categories (of either similar or different status), known as horizontal segregation (Hakim, 1979), is demonstrated by the fact that over a half of all women work in just three occupations:

- clerical and secretarial;
- personal and protective services, such as nursing, catering, cleaning, hairdressing;
- sales occupations.

These occupations are also those with the greatest numbers of part-time workers, in which women outnumber men, with the poorest wage levels and conditions of employment, and where the demand for female labour has been greatest. Moreover, they are becoming more feminised as more women enter these already female-dominated occupations.

At the same time, more women are entering male-dominated occupations and appear to be becoming more integrated into the labour market (Rubery and Fagan, 1993). They have increased their share of higher-level jobs as a result both of the expansion of these occupations as a consequence of organisational restructuring and of technical change, as well as increasing levels of qualifications amongst women, their continuity of employment and proximity to employment opportunities in the south-east. Thus women are beginning to account for a higher proportion of employment in managerial and professional occupations: for instance, between 1981 and 1990 the proportion of women in managerial occupations grew from 22 to 28 per cent.

Few women, however, reach the top jobs in management or the professions. In part, this is because of the nature of organisations and their tendency to reproduce, through a variety of processes, gendered power relations and prevailing notions of masculinity (Cockburn, 1991). So women experience vertical segregation whereby men and women in the same occupation attain different hierarchical levels. Hence a recent study found one in four junior managers in Britain were women, whereas at senior management level the proportion of women was down to 1 or 2 per cent (Summers, 1991). Similar examples are found throughout most professions: women account for only 12 per cent of partners in law firms, 15 per cent of medical consultants and 3 per cent of university professors or principal lecturers (Rice, 1991; Summers, 1991).

Women's entry into previously male-dominated jobs does not necessarily herald a decline in segregation. Often these changes involve transformations in the organisation of these occupations, leading to deskilling and/or downgrading of the pay, status and/or career opportunities associated with the occupation. As Rubery and Fagan comment:

> Evidence of desegregation may in fact be an indicator of a new pattern of segregation and not evidence of a trend towards integration and equality: moreover decreased horizontal segregation . . . may in fact reduce rather than expand opportunities for vertical mobility, thereby increasing segregation . . . at least within occupational areas. (1994: 30)

These two contrasting developments of increasing feminisation of certain jobs, on the one hand, and increasing integration of women into higher level jobs, on the other, suggest a growing polarisation between women in the labour market. In other words, there is developing greater diversity and inequalities between groups of women in the labour market which point to their heterogeneity.

These trends are likely to continue in the future. The greatest employment growth is anticipated in managerial and professional occupations and women are expected to share in this occupational growth. For example, women are expected to be 38 per cent of managers and administrators, 41 per cent of professional and 53 per cent of associated professional and technical employees by the year 2000 (Wilson, 1994).

Pay

Following the introduction of the 1970 Equal Pay Act women's average hourly earnings (excluding overtime) rose from 64 per cent of men's to 74 per cent. Between 1977 and 1987 there was no significant improvement in women's pay, despite a broadening of the legislation in 1984. Since 1987 women's pay has increased relative to men's and now stands at 79 per cent of men's (Employment Department, 1993c). These recent gains in women's pay are probably related to the rise in full-time work rates and decline in levels of occupational segregation.

Women, as well as earning less than men, are concentrated in the lowest-paid jobs. Overall, three times as many women as men working full-time are in low-paid jobs. However, women in full-time manual jobs are five times more likely than men to earn low wages – 30 per cent as against 6 per cent.

The undervaluing of women's paid work is associated with three inter-related factors:

- widespread occupational segregation by gender;
- gender discrimination in the ways in which jobs are graded and paid;
- differences in the labour supply and labour market conditions for men and women which allow these differences to be perpetuated.

Barriers to employment and policy responses

Key barriers to employment

The above analysis of women's changing position in the labour market as well as occupational structures suggests that they face a range of barriers in gaining employment and better jobs. These include the following:

- Structural barriers within the labour market, such as the demand for labour and the growth of certain types of jobs especially part-time jobs in a limited number of occupations which leads to gender occupational segregation and contributes to women's low pay relative to men's.
- Organisational barriers encountered through employers' policies and practices such as those maintaining vertical occupational segregation and the gender division of labour in occupations and organisations. The lack of part-time opportunities in managerial jobs, flexible working arrangements, and 'family-friendly' policies persist despite the increasing proportion of working mothers.
- Institutional barriers include, for instance, access to qualifications and training for different skill levels. The lack of training and qualifications prevent women from moving up the occupational hierarchy into better and more highly paid jobs. Moreover, as we have seen, they inhibit the participation of lone parents while also disadvantaging women returners and those women taking time out of the labour market to have children.
- Attitudinal barriers of employers, for instance those related to gender stereotypes, affect employers' willingness to recruit and promote women with children or women of child-bearing age into their organisation or into certain types of jobs. And women's own attitudes may affect their behaviour in the labour market, for example in terms of the importance they attach to paid work in comparison to their family.

How has the government, in recent years, responded to women's changing position in the labour market and the barriers they encounter? How have they translated these barriers into tangible and concrete issues which are amenable to policy development? Before answering these questions let us first examine the overall thrust of the government's labour market policies in recent years.

Labour market policies

One of the hallmarks of the Conservative government is that it abandoned a commitment to full employment (however defined) which had been a focus of government economic and social policy in post-war Britain. The current Conservative government sees the promotion of a flexible, efficient and competitive labour market as central to achieving sustained, non-inflationary growth. It believes that this can be achieved through a process of deregulation. According to its philosophy, inflexible and over-regulated labour markets deter employers from taking on new employees, prevent employers and employees from agreeing the flexible work patterns they both want and damage job creation. Overall, therefore, it adopts a non-interventionist and voluntarist approach to employment policies rather than active labour market policies. It believes in the supremacy of the market. Employers and employees should be free to determine working relationships, employment conditions and working arrangements.

According to a recent government White Paper *Competitiveness: Helping business to win* (1994), the main objectives of its strategy for improving the working of the labour market since 1979 have been the following:

- to maximise the effective supply of labour and competition for jobs;
- to enhance the quality of the workforce;
- to encourage good employment practices;
- to improve industrial relations;
- ●RI1to maintain a fair framework for individual employment rights, while minimising costs to employers;
- to reform and encourage change in wage bargaining arrangements.

Where do women fit in this overall strategy and how have women fared as a result of this strategy? It is not possible, in the bounds of this chapter, to discuss all the different elements of government policy in meeting these objectives. Instead we shall concentrate on just the first two objectives. Policies aimed at maximising the supply of women workers have concentrated on getting rid of unfair discrimination; childcare policies; and maternity provision. Those aimed at enhancing the quality of the workforce have focused on improving the skill levels of the workforce primarily through education[6] and training. Let us now examine these policies in turn.

Sex equality legislation

The 1975 Sex Discrimination Act is the main legislation specifically dealing with women's employment and training opportunities and other non-contractual aspects of employment, while the 1970 Equal Pay Act covers contractual aspects. The legislation is overseen by the Equal Opportunities Commission which has certain limited powers to investigate unequal treatment.

The Sex Discrimination Act is a blanket piece of legislation aimed at outlawing both direct and indirect discrimination in employment, education, the provision of goods and services and advertising. It also outlaws discrimination on the basis of marital status in access to jobs, recruitment, selection and opportunities for training, promotion or transfer and dismissal. Only under restricted circumstances does it allow positive action.

It is very difficult to establish a conclusive causal relationship between this Act and its effect on women's employment. It is open to debate whether legislation can change attitudes or just reflects existing attitudes. Moreover, in recent years, the impact of the legislation has been dwarfed by more far-reaching Directives and changes coming from the European Community.

Most of the growth in women's employment can be attributed to changes both in the demand for labour and in the structure of the labour market rather than the legislation. The legislation, however, may have improved the efficiency of the labour market by eradicating the most blatant forms of discrimination, thus increasing the supply of women workers. It may have encouraged more liberal attitudes towards women's role, their entry into further and higher education, and their subsequent entry into the professions and traditionally male-dominated higher-level jobs. The legislation's lack of more substantive impact can be related, in part, to its inherent limitations[7] and, in part, to its underpinning ideology and model of inequality upon which it is based (see below). As a result, it has failed to deal with the underlying reasons for discrimination, including the role of women in society and the interaction of the family and the labour market. Nor has it been able to overcome occupational segregation and its roots in the sexual division of labour or the forces that make it so attractive in the pursuit of profitability.

Under the Equal Pay Act a woman must be paid the same as a man if she is doing broadly similar work, work which has been rated as equivalent by a job evaluation study or work which is of equal value in terms of effort, skill and decision making. The latter condition was only introduced in 1984 as a result of the principles embedded in Article 119 of the Treaty of Rome and the European Community's 1975 Directive on equal pay.

This legislation has had a mixed impact on women's pay (see above). Initially it positively affected pay differentials between the sexes (Zabalza and Tzannatos, 1985) but more recent changes in differentials are unlikely to be attributable to the legislation (Hakim, 1993). In addition, the legislation has failed to impact on women's low pay. Indeed, women's low pay has been adversely affected by another objective in the government's labour market strategy: namely, its reform of wage-bargaining arrangements. In particular, it abolished the Wages Council, which set minimum rates of pay. Three-quarters of all workers covered by the Wages Council were women (MacLennan, 1980) and thus women have been especially affected. Overall, however, the legislation has been unable to tackle women's low pay because it leaves untouched the problem of occupational segregation and women's concentration in low-paying part-time jobs.

Childcare policies

It is well established that the lack of affordable childcare is a major impediment to women's participation in both employment and training. The government, however, has no coherent childcare policy. Nor has it implemented legislation on childcare except to regulate standards of provision. Its overall philosophy is that childcare is the responsibility of individual mothers (not parents) and can be supplied through the market. It offers few fiscal or financial incentives to encourage employer provision despite calls upon employers to provide facilities.

Recently, however, the government has introduced two childcare policies aimed at increasing the supply of women workers and improving work incentives. In December 1992 the government announced a new initiative, with a budget of £45 million over three years, to encourage out-of-school childcare. It aims 'to help parents enter or participate more fully in work or training' (Employment Department/Kids Club Network, n.d.) by improving the quantity and quality of childcare available outside school hours and during school holidays. The grants administered locally by Training and Enterprise Councils (see below) are designed to provide 'pump-priming' money to develop a variety of schemes in conjunction with employers, local authorities and schools. Over 1,000 new places were created in the first six months, with a further 1,100 in development. It is anticipated that the funds will help create 50,000 out-of-school childcare places (Evidence from the Employment Department to the Employment Select Committee: Provision for Working Mothers, 1994). This initiative is concerned about increasing the actual supply of childcare provision but the issue of its cost and affordability remain untouched. Moreover, the scale of provision will be very limited given the overall budget.

In the 1993 November Budget another measure was announced to help low-income families which enables them to offset £40 a week of their childcare costs against their earnings.[8] It aims to boost the supply of women in the labour market by increasing incentives for families to find and remain in employment.[9] Only families using formal (i.e. registered childminders or nursery) rather than informal (i.e. friends and relatives) care will be able to claim the disregard for children under 11 years. Those on Family Credit will receive a maximum of £28 once the effects of the benefit's taper is taken into account. It is estimated that the measure will help 100,000 people on low earnings and a further 50,000 to take up paid work (Cm. 2563, 1994). Initial criticism has focused on the inadequacy of the level of earnings disregard, the restriction to formal childcare costs, the lack of cover for those in receipt of income support and, above all, its availability to limited categories of mothers.

Maternity provision

As a result of the trade Union Reform and Employment Rights Act 1993, from October 1994 all women qualify for a minimum of 14 weeks' maternity leave with a right to return to work, irrespective of their length of service or hours of work. In addition, women who have been continuously employed for 26 weeks are eligible for statutory maternity pay set at 90 per cent of earnings for the first six weeks and £52.50 for the remaining 12 weeks.[10]

Interestingly, these improvements arise from a European Council Directive 92/85/EEC on health and safety, known as the Protection of Pregnant Women at Work, yet they have been promoted by the government as measures to help women wanting to combine a career with family responsibilities, hence increasing their supply. The changes have been criticised, however, because the amount of leave is too short; the levels of pay too little; the legislative framework for maternity rights remains complicated for both employees and employers alike; and some women are still excluded from some of the provisions. More significantly, the government is requiring employers (except small employers) to meet some of the additional cost of improvements to maternity pay. Ultimately, this might damage women's employment opportunities as some employers may be put off employing women of child-bearing age. Thus, rather than increasing the supply of women workers, the legislation in fact may reduce that supply.

Government training policies

There is no government legislation or explicit policies specifically aimed at women's training. Nor does the government have a national education and training strategy which explicitly takes account of women's needs except in acknowledging their growing importance in the labour market.

The government adopts a non-interventionist approach to training. It sees employers rather than the state as having the key responsibility for training. It relies upon the market to meet training needs and upon individuals to pursue their own careers. However, it recognises it has a role in providing training for those with no access to employers' training, namely the long-term unemployed.

The government has taken a proactive role in encouraging the take-up of vocational training and improving standards. It has introduced training initiatives such as the National Targets for Education and Training and Investors in People and set up agencies with responsibility for developing the direction and content of vocational training, such as the National Council for Vocational Qualifications. Together these aim to raise the skills of the workforce as a whole, but their efforts are not directed specifically at women.

Training and Enterprise Councils

Following the 1973 Employment and Training Act, all government training programmes were delivered and administered centrally through the Manpower Services Commission and subsequently through the Training Enterprise and Education Directorate of the Department of Employment. The 1988 government White Paper *Employment for the 1990s*, however, introduced a new national network of local employer-led Training and Enterprise Councils (TECs) in England and Wales and Local Enterprise Companies (LECs) in Scotland. These agencies have been responsible for delivering and developing the government's training and enterprise programmes since 1990.

TECs and LECs now have a pre-eminent role in delivering public-funded vocational training based on the skill needs of the local labour market and therefore have an important role in the pursuit of equal opportunities. They do not provide training directly but make contracts with local training providers such as colleges, private trainers and employers. Their funding from central government and their payments to training providers are output-related. It is dependent on participants meeting certain targets, such as getting a job or vocational qualification.

TECs and equal opportunities

TECs have a contractual obligation to abide by the relevant sex equality legislation (see above), to incorporate equal opportunity principles in all their activities and to ensure that training providers promote equal opportunities.

A recent formal investigation into TECs by the Equal Opportunities Commission 1993), however, has highlighted the shortcoming with TECs' pursuit of equal opportunities: for instance, only 58 per cent of TECs had undertaken or were about to undertake special initiatives for women. The investigation concluded that TECs needed to be much more proactive in helping and promoting equal opportunities.

Government training programmes

The government's main contribution to training provision has been training programmes (delivered by TECs) aimed at the unemployed. These consist of Youth Training (YT) and Training for Work (TFW), which replaced Employment Training (ET) in April 1993. These programmes account for only a small proportion of all training activity. In 1991 almost nine-tenths of training occurred outside of YT and ET. These schemes, however, are extremely important for the most disadvantaged groups in the labour market and they are of obvious concern in the context of this chapter.

Youth Training

Youth Training aims to provide broad vocational education and training mainly for 16–18-year-olds and in March 1994 287,200 people were involved (Employment Department, 1994). Priority is given to young people under the age of 18 who have left full-time education and are not employed. YT programmes are usually a mixture of work experience and off-the-job training and must lead to a National Vocational Qualification (NVQ)[11] Level 2 or equivalent. Young men are considerably more likely to join YT than young women. Women represent about 40 per cent of trainees but 52 per cent of the unemployed (International Labour Office (ILO) definition) in this age group. The majority of these women undertake training in traditionally female areas such as clerical and administrative work (Clarke, 1991).

Despite a formal commitment to equal opportunities YT and its predecessor (Youth Training Scheme – YTS) have had little impact on occupational gender segregation. As Cockburn's (1987) study showed, there are strong links between sex segregation in training and occupational segregation in the labour market as a whole. Culturally determined definitions of skill along with cultural norms and ideology associated with masculinity and femininity largely determined the type of training young men and women pursued. YTS failed to enable women to cross into 'gender-contrary' areas of training and, as a result, it helped to perpetuate occupational segregation rather than ameliorate it.

Data on YT leavers for 1992/3 reveal other significant differences in young women and men's experiences of YT (Murray, 1994) but cannot explain these differences.

- More young women (61 per cent) left YT early compared to men (55 per cent).
- Just over a half of young women (52 per cent) entered employment after leaving YT compared to 48 per cent of young men.
- A similar proportion of young women and men (47 per cent) gained a qualification or credit on leaving YT but the level of qualification women gained was lower compared to young men.[12]

Training for Work

Training for Work was introduced in April 1993 and replaces Employment Training. It is the major programme available for long-term unemployed adults. It aims to help them to find jobs and to improve their work-related skills by providing training and structured work activity in line with their assessed needs.

Training for Work is open to those aged 18–59 who have been *registered* unemployed for 26 weeks or more, with priority given to those unemployed at least a year and unemployed people with disabilities. Certain groups do not have to have been unemployed for 26 weeks and they include lone parents in receipt of the social security benefit or income support and women returners.

Although the eligibility conditions for TFW are more advantageous to women compared with its predecessor ET, it is likely that some women will continue to miss out on training opportunities. First, women are much less likely to register as unemployed compared with men because registration is linked to the receipt of social security benefits and unemployment benefit, in particular. Women, especially married women, those who have worked part-time or want part-time work and those with dependants, are often not eligible for unemployment benefit. Consequently, they do not register as unemployed and therefore, in practice, may be denied access to TFW. Secondly, women are particularly under-represented among the registered long-term unemployed because of the operation of the social security system and yet the long-term unemployed are a key priority group. Thus TFW indirectly discriminates against women because of its eligibility criteria.

Women also are disadvantaged by the way training through TECs is funded (EOC, 1993). Output-related funding acts as a major disincentive in the recruitment of some trainees, especially women returners. There is potential for discrimination against lone parents who are eligible for childcare support because they are more expensive to train. Finally, there is a lack of part-time training opportunities, in part because such courses tend to be less cost-effective than full-time courses.

Women are also likely to miss out on TFW because of the way training provision is organised. Participation on a part-time basis is at the discretion of the TEC or provider and is not guaranteed. Like ET, allowances to meet childcare costs are discretionary and can be given to lone parents only. Both the level of allowance and the eligibility criteria are at the discretion of the TEC and provider.

Given TECs' record on equal-opportunities and funding arrangements for TFW, TFW's eligibility criteria and the lack of guaranteed childcare and part-time training, it is not surprising that of the 150,000 people on TFW in March 1994 only 33 per cent were women. Data on ET for 1992/3 reveal that more women (41 per cent) gained employment on leaving the scheme than men (30 per cent). More women (43 per cent) than men (36 per cent) gained a qualification or credit, however, they gained lower-level qualifications than their male counterparts (Murray, 1994).[13] Hence, these women, like their younger colleagues on YT, are only being equipped to take jobs in limited occupations and at relatively low levels.

The limitations of policy

Nature of the limitations

It is too early to judge what the long-term effects of the more recent government policies will be upon women's position in the labour market. We can question, however, how adequate they are in meeting women's needs given their changing position in the labour market. To what extent will they increase the supply of women workers and improve their skills? To what extent are they likely to impact on ocupational segregation and women's concentration in low-skilled and low-paid jobs? The evidence so far suggests that these policies are unlikely to have a radical effect on these dynamics. Indeed, there is evidence that points to quite the opposite – that they will perpetuate and maintain women's disadvantaged position in the labour market.

The childcare provisions introduced are very limited and do not represent a comprehensive childcare policy. What is required is a national childcare policy and action plan that meet the needs of all working mothers. Similarly, as we have seen, there are no comprehensive policies for women returners despite their rise in number and the problems they face. Nor is there an overall strategy for women's training. Women's access to publicly funded training is restricted while the training provided does not take into consideration their particular needs. This lack of training strategy aimed specifically at women means that women will continue to be at a disadvantage in comparison to men.

The piecemeal and fragmented nature of government policies means that they are likely to have only a very limited impact on women in the labour market. What is required is a more radical and holistic approach. Such a strategy would need policies that dealt with the following:

Acquisition and re-acquisition of skills. The main factors include:

- women's limited access to training to gain the skills and qualifications required in the labour market;

- access to training which depends too heavily on being employed to provide such training – women without jobs or with only poor jobs do not have effective access to training to enable them to get jobs or better jobs;
- limited access to training which supplies a supportive learning environment and acknowledges their specific requirements.

Deployment of skills. Women encounter structural constraints on taking up training or when entering employment, after having obtained suitable training, such as adequate childcare provision to make it possible, good contractual conditions (especially regarding part-time work) to make it beneficial and open occupational structures, free of segmentation, to make it sustainable.

Rewards for skills. Discriminatory payment and grading systems and employer practices which undermine the initial returns from employment and training, bias household decisions in favour of men working and reduce incentives to build up more human capital on which to base further career development.

Factors limiting policy

These above proposals assume, however, that employment and social policies can radically impact on women's position in the labour market. They are based on a range of assumptions which need to be questioned. Firstly, the demand for legislative change supposes that the state is a proper and neutral arbiter. Legislation, however, can be manipulated to the advantage of powerful representatives of capitalism and patriarchy. For example, protective legislation for women has often been used by men to exclude them from the labour market and the new maternity legislation may be used in a similar way. Secondly, legislation can have unintended consequences which are contrary to its stated aims and objectives. For instance, when the equal pay legislation was originally introduced some employers tried to avoid equal pay claims by reorganising their workforce so men and women were not doing similar work. As a result, occupational segregation at the level of the firm actually increased. Thirdly, legislation can act in conflicting ways. Despite the government's commitment to equal pay and improving women's position in the labour market, it has introduced policies which are likely to increase inequalities rather than ameliorate them. The abolition of the Wages Councils is a case in point.

Implicit in many policies aimed at reducing inequalities is the premise that if women improved their human capital through gaining more qualifications and experience then occupational segregation would be reduced. Such an approach sees the main problems as lying with women and their lack of qualifications. It is a highly individualistic stance and ignores the complex ways in which occupational segregation is both structured and perpetuated.

Indeed policies aimed at lifting barriers and promoting equal opportunities are oversimplistic and overoptimistic. The ideas informing such strategies are preoccupied with attitudes, stereotypes, choices and underachievement. They are based on a narrow view of inequality which underpins most policy provision including the sex equality legislation. This view assumes that inequalities arise because women are subject to prejudice resulting from stereotypical beliefs about their characteristics *as a group*. The solution is, firstly, to change employers' attitudes and, secondly, to get employers to use procedures which force them to look at job candidates as *individuals*, judged on their own merits. In this way problems of equal access can be overcome.

An alternative, broader view of inequality goes beyond seeing the problem in terms of equal access and stereotypical assumptions. It begins by addressing the current structure of employment aiming to analyse and counter the ways in which occupational segregation is perpetuated through social and cultural structures. It acknowledges past discrimination and disadvantage outside of the workplace. In particular, it recognises that not everyone starts at the same point and so disadvantage will continue unless steps are made to compensate for past disadvantage. Thus it incorporates a notion of differential need while recognising that women are not a homogeneous group. Above all, it is concerned with outcomes.

Because most policies are based on the former narrow view of inequality, they give insufficient consideration to the structures of inequality and the processes by which those with power and status resist attempts by women to better their labour market position. They overlook the way the social structure, the economy, the labour process and dynamics in the workplace give rise to inequalities. As a result, they fail to acknowledge the sexual division of labour inside and outside of the family and the relations between women's paid and unpaid work. Above all, they ignore the structural constraints on women arising from capitalism and patriarchy and the way these forces shape women's position in the labour market.

Notes

1. Unless otherwise stated, the statistics in the remainder of this chapter are drawn from data from the Labour Force Survey and cover Great Britain.
2. In 1979 38 per cent of all lone parents received supplementary benefit, by 1991 the proportion receiving income support had risen to 70 per cent.
3. Forty-three per cent of lone parents have no qualification compared to 32 per cent of married mothers; around a third of lone parents say they have never worked before becoming a lone parent (Bartholomew *et al.*, 1992); 44 per cent of non-employed lone parents say they would return to work sooner if there were childcare available (Bradshaw and Millar, 1991).
4. There are distinct limitations to these labour market statistics in measuring the labour market activities of ethnic minorities. For instance, a sizeable number of women fall uneasily between ethnic minority and ethnic majority status and the Labour Force Survey may under-represent ethnic minority women's work. For a fuller discussion see, for example, Nanton (1992) and Jones (1993).

5. These figures incorporate the standard ILO definition of the unemployed which is those who work, are available to start work in two weeks and have looked for work within the previous four weeks plus those who have not recently looked for work.

6. Issues concerning education are not discussed as these are examined elsewhere in this volume.

7. The legislation has been criticised for being too individualistic; for being too complex and costly to implement in practice; for relying on individuals to bring cases forward and not incorporating the notion of 'class actions'; and for not advocating positive discrimination.

8. It applies to families on family credit, disability working allowance, housing benefit and council tax benefit and will come into force in October 1994.

9. Another major plank of government policy aimed at increasing women's work incentives is the social security benefit family credit. For a discussion of this benefit see Marsh and McKay (1993b), McKay and Marsh (1994), Callender *et al.* (forthcoming).

10. For details of the current provision and the changes see IDS, March 1994.

11. National Vocational Qualifications are new vocational qualifications which were introduced in the late 1980s. Unlike previous qualifications, they are based on performance and nationally agreed standards and competences which reflect activities in the workplace. For more information of them and their take-up and usage by employers see Callender *et al.* (1993).

12. Of all the women gaining a qualification 83 per cent gained an NVQ at Level 1 or 2 and the remaining 17 per cent achieved a Level 3 or 4, while the equivalent figures for young men were 69 per cent and 31 per cent.

13. Of those women gaining an NVQ on leaving ET, 96 per cent achieved a Level 1 or 2 and 4 per cent an NVQ at a higher level. The equivalent proportions for men were 84 per cent and 16 per cent (Murray, 1994).

4   *Women, poverty and social security*

Jane Millar

Women outnumber men among those living in poverty, their chances of being poor are higher and they stay poor for longer. Thus women have a greater incidence, a higher risk and longer durations of poverty compared with men. Over the past decade poverty and inequality have increased very substantially in the United Kingdom. However the risk of poverty does not fall equally: some people never experience poverty, for others poverty is a short episode quickly recovered from, while for others poverty is a long-term experience affecting all aspects of their lives. It is this last group whose numbers have been rising so sharply in recent years and increasingly it is families with dependent children who are to be found among these long-term poor. Motherhood – whether in a two-parent or a lone-parent family – is thus increasingly associated with poverty and, because women with children are usually responsible for both housework and housekeeping, these mothers also bear the responsibility of trying to make ends meet and protect their families from the worst effects of poverty.

Poverty is clearly a women's issue but it is only relatively recently that research attention has focused specifically on the gender dimensions of poverty (Land, 1983a; Glendinning and Millar, 1987). In part, this is because women's poverty has become much more visible in recent years, for example among the rapidly rising numbers of lone mothers (Millar, 1987); in part, also, the interest reflects the influence of feminist ideas and research, especially in-depth research on the day-to-day lives of women in their families (Pahl, 1980; Graham, 1987). A focus on gender often starts by 'adding women in' to existing approaches and data and thus one of the aims of the initial work on women and poverty was to find data on poverty which allowed comparisons to be made between men and women. It rapidly became obvious, however, that this was not just a simple statistical exercise but that it fundamentally called into question the ways in which poverty was both conceptualised and measured. Analysing the gender dimensions of poverty thus meant rethinking the concept itself, not simply 'adding women in' but 'revising the concept' (Millar and Glendinning, 1989; Jenkins, 1991). The first part of this chapter provides a review of these arguments.

Women often earn their poverty through low-paid jobs (as Claire Callender discusses in Chapter 3) but, in addition, women are very often dependent on the state for all or most of their incomes. There were, for example, in 1993 about 6.5 million women pensioners and about 2.7 million women claiming income support (DSS, 1993). Women outnumber men as recipients of all the main benefits, with the exceptions of unemployment benefit, invalidity benefit and industrial injury disablement benefit (Lister, 1992). Women also receive benefits on behalf of others, especially children, and there are about 7 million women receiving child benefit as well as about half a million receiving family credit. In addition many women live in families where their husband is receiving benefit for the family as a whole. Almost 1 million women were living on income support claimed by their partners in 1992 (DSS, 1993) and Esam and Berthoud (1991) have calculated that a social security benefit of some kind is paid to around 3.7 million married men in respect of their wives. Up until fairly recently the social security system directly discriminated against married women, who were not entitled to claim benefits on the same basis as men. This direct discrimination has largely been removed, with the European Commission and the European Court of Justice playing an important part in enforcing commitments to equal treatment (Millar, 1989; Whitting, 1992). However this formal equality does not necessarily ensure equality in outcome, with women's actual access to social security benefits, especially social insurance benefits, still more restricted than that of men (Pascall, 1986; Lister, 1992). The second main section of this chapter examines these issues and concludes with a brief discussion of ways in which the benefit system could be reformed to meet the needs of women more adequately.

Women and poverty: extent, nature, causes and consequences

Official statistics fight shy of the word 'poverty' and tend to focus instead on 'low-income families' or 'households below the average'. As poverty has increased through the 1980s so the debate about the definition of poverty has intensified: are families living on benefits actually living in poverty? To what extent is poverty caused by bad management rather than incomes that are too low to meet needs? Are low incomes indicative of poverty or simply of inequality? However, although the interpretation of the statistics may be open to debate, the picture that is painted, from a number of different sources, is quite clear: the numbers of people living on very low incomes have increased significantly. For example, Department of Social Security figures show that the number of people living in households with incomes of less than half the average, after meeting housing costs, was 5 million (9 per cent of the population) in 1979; by 1991/2 this had risen to 13.9 million or 25 per cent of the population (DSS, 1994). Goodman and Webb (1994), in their analysis of the distribution of income over thirty years, show that it has been in the 1980s in particular that inequalities in income have widened dramatically. Jenkins (1994) points to increasing inequalities in wages as the key factor driving this.

Unfortunately, however, these data are only of very limited use in tracing trends in women's poverty. The main reason for this is that, in all these studies, poverty is measured on either a household or a family basis rather than on an individual basis.[1] So, taking the 'households below average income' figures as a measure, the figure of 13.9 million poor people actually means that there are 13.9 million people living in households in which the total household income, adjusted for household size, falls below the poverty line. Thus, although it is individuals who are counted, the measure of poverty used is an aggregate and not an individual measure. There are some good reasons why aggregate measures are used: some people, especially children, have no incomes of their own but are supported by other family members; people who live together do share living standards to some degree; people sharing can live more cheaply than people living alone (Millar and Glendinning, 1987). Thus family (or household) income is assumed to be a better indicator of living standards, and hence poverty, than individual measures of income.

The concept of 'family income' is a construction, however, created by combining all the sources of income coming into the family into a single measure. The concept of family income thus rests on two key assumptions. The first is that everyone in the family shares equally in that income and thus that they all share the same standard of living – they are all either poor or non-poor and, if they are poor, they are all poor to the same degree. Secondly, it is assumed that the source of the various components that make up the family income is irrelevant; all money coming into the home is equally available to be used in the same way. However, neither assumption is supported by the empirical evidence and the concept of family income thus serves to obscure gender differences in the extent and experience of poverty.

The concept of family income

Looking first at the assumption of equal sharing, studies on the distribution of resources within households have found that the ways in which people who live together deal with their money is much more complicated than this. Pahl (1980), in her pioneering work on this subject, identified four main systems of money management. She drew up this categorisation on the basis of in-depth interviews with a relatively small sample, but more recently Vogler and Pahl (1993) have applied this, in a slightly more extended form, to a large sample of couples of working age. This gives an indication of the prevalence of the different management systems among couples (as yet this work has not been extended to families or households more generally).

The *female whole wage system* describes a situation where the man hands over all his wages to the woman, who takes complete responsibility for all housekeeping. About 26 per cent of all couples use this system. Less common is the *male whole wage system*, where the man both controls and manages all the money, used by 10 per cent. The *housekeeping allowance system* is where the man pays some of the major commitments such as housing costs and large bills and gives the woman an allowance to meet the day-to-day households costs. About 12 per cent of all couples fall into this group. These systems are more likely to be used when there is only one wage earner. Among two-earner couples the *independent management* system means both keep their incomes separate and take separate responsibility for the various financial commitments. Only 2 per cent of couples use this system. Finally, there is the *pooling system*, in which all the money is put into a common pool and spent, as appropriate, by either member of the couple. About half of all couples say they use this system, but Vogler and Pahl argue that this system needs to be further sub-divided into three distinct categories, depending on who has the final say in decisions about expenditure: the *male-managed pool* (15 per cent), the *female-managed pool* (15 per cent) and the *joint pool* (20 per cent).

Thus it is clear that, although couples do share their incomes in various ways, it is not correct to assume that all the money coming into the family is available in the same way to all family members. Only about two in every ten couples have the sort of joint pool that is assumed in the concept of family income. In addition, it is clear from these studies on money management within families that the source of income is important in determining how money is perceived and can be spent. Although women's earnings are forming an increasing proportion of family income (Land, 1994; Machin and Waldfogel, 1994), the idea, or ideal, of the man as the breadwinner remains very strong. The fact that the man earns the money gives him greater control over how it should be spent and makes it legitimate for him to retain some part of the total income as personal spending money or 'pocket money'. Burgoyne (1990: 662), in her analysis of how perceived ownership of money plays a part in its use among married couples, concludes that:

> In our society, an individual has certain rights of ownership and control over money s/he has earned or inherited. Marital ideology, on the other hand, currently poses a challenge to such rights. . . . Pooling money in a joint account may remove the overt labels of ownership, but the source of that money may retain a powerful influence on the minds of both partners, an influence which is not consciously admitted, yet which may be reflected in the way both partners treat what is, in theory, a joint resource.

Even the joint pool, therefore, does not eradicate the concepts of 'his' or 'her' money. For non-employed women the lack of any money 'of their own' is therefore seen as putting constraints on what they can and cannot do in spending money. Child benefit is highly valued by such women, as being their own source of income separate from their partners' (Walker *et al.*, 1994). Earnings are even better in terms of giving independence, although in practice women's earnings tend to get spent on family needs and women in low-income families rarely keep a designated sum of money for themselves (Pahl, 1989). Moreover, as Vogler and Pahl (1993) show, couples with the man in full-time work and the woman either not employed or in part-time work (the most common pattern among families with children) are the most likely to use male-managed systems, and the women, although perhaps responsible for day-to-day spending, have little real control and power.

The concept of a family income is not simply a research tool; it also has an ideological function as part of the construction of the family as belonging to the 'private' sphere, where it is not the business of policy to penetrate. As Dilnot *et al.* (1984: 112) put it, 'the distribution of income between husband and wife is a matter for them rather than for the government.' Alongside the ideology of the family as an egalitarian unit this means that issues of intra-family income distribution often only become visible when families break down. Studies of lone mothers show that typically about a third of them say that they are financially better off by themselves than when they were with their partners. This is not because their income is higher – lone motherhood almost always means a fall in income – but because the money is all theirs to control and spend and one of the good things about lone motherhood is this independence from male financial control (Bradshaw and Millar, 1991). The ending of marriage also exposes family income as a myth in another way. In the divorce courts and now in the Child Support Agency there is no presumption that the total family income belongs to *all* the family and should be divided between them. Instead the man's earnings are seen as belonging to him and the objective is to decide how much he can contribute towards his children, after meeting his own needs (and those of his second family, if he has one). The women have no entitlement to a share in this income except in their role as carer of the children. The tension between the dual function of wages, as both a reward for individual work and as a means of subsistence, is especially apparent when these claims clash, as they do when families separate.

Thus the assumption of pooling, central to family-based measures of income poverty, does not represent what actually happens in practice and this means that the extent of poverty among women is underestimated in conventional studies. To examine how far this is the case Davies and Joshi (1994) have estimated two sets of poverty rates for men and women based on two different assumptions about income sharing. Counting those whose incomes are in the bottom fifth of the income distribution as poor and using the conventional pooled income measure, they estimate that 15 per cent of married men and married women were in poverty in 1986 (the figures are, of course, the same for men and women because it is assumed that they each have the same share of income). Then they take the extreme opposite assumption, that there is 'minimal' sharing which means that the couple share housing costs but nothing else. On this measure 52 per cent of married women were under the poverty line compared with only 11 per cent of married men. The minimal sharing assumption is, of course, also unrealistic but nevertheless these figures show that about half of all married women do not have, *in their own right*, an income sufficient to keep them out of poverty.

Evason (1991) uses a different methodology to make the same point. She argues that poverty should be measured in relation to independent access to income, which would 'come closer to conveying the reality of women's material position' than aggregate measures can (p. 65; see also Jenkins, 1991; Glendinning and Millar, 1992). Using Northern Ireland data, Evason counts up the three main groups of women with access to little or no income in their own right (non-employed married women, employed but low-paid women, non-employed single women in receipt of benefits). On this basis, she estimates that 'three-quarters of adult women in Northern Ireland do not have access in their own right to income above the level of means-tested benefits' (1991: 66). Esam and Berthoud (1991) similarly calculate that, in 1991/2, about 4.6 million women in Britain had independent incomes of less than £25 per week compared with only 0.4 million men.

Standards of living and unpaid work

So far the discussion has concentrated on income-based measures of poverty. In these measures the focus is very much on 'inputs', on the resources that are available to maintain a particular standard of living. However, it has also been argued that more attention should be paid to 'outputs' – to the actual standard of living that people have, as measured, for example, by their access to assets and their patterns of consumption (Ringen, 1988; Callan *et al.*, 1993). This formulation of poverty, however, also raises gender issues. Household measures of consumption and assets, like household measures of income, assume all family members share equally in these assets. But studies of within-household consumption patterns show the same picture as the studies of within-household income distribution: men tend to be privileged consumers, for example, of food, of cars, of space, of heat (Millar and Glendinning, 1989). In addition the unpaid work that women do in the home plays a key part in determining the living standards of the family. First women are responsible for the bulk of the domestic work – the shopping, cooking, cleaning – and it is their skills in these areas that determine the living standards of the family. Secondly, women often cut back on their own needs in order to try and protect their families, husbands and especially children, from the worst effects of poverty. Thirdly, in poor families, women are more likely to be responsible for managing the money. Management of money in these circumstances is a difficult chore rather than a source of power and, probably not surprisingly, women in poor families report higher levels of stress than men (Bradshaw and Holmes, 1989).

Thus the unpaid work that women do in the home is central to how they, and other family members, experience poverty. A recent study of 74 poor families, 34 couples and 40 lone parents highlights the way in which living in poverty means a constant struggle to make ends meet (Kempson *et al.*, 1994). These families, far from being inefficient managers or work-shy scroungers, were continually seeking ways either to improve their income (find work, get overtime, claim benefits and so on) or to manage what they had as best they could. The researchers identified two main management strategies. On the one hand, there are those who try to manage by juggling with their bills and debts. This is very stressful and extracts a high cost in terms of constant worry and ill health. On the other hand, there are those who try to manage by keeping a very tight control over all their expenditure. The costs of this strategy are a sacrifice of material welfare and social participation. All those living in these poor families suffered because no matter how much juggling they did or how careful they were there was simply not enough money to go round. But much of the stress and strain of poverty fell upon the women, either as lone mothers or as the ones responsible for trying to budget on such low incomes. Thus poor women, including lone mothers, have high levels of ill health, both physical and mental (Popay and Jones, 1990; Payne, 1991). Using smoking to control stress and to gain some individual time and space is common among poor women (Graham, 1993b; Marsh and McKay, 1994) but this is a strategy very damaging to health in the longer run.

Without women's paid work there would be many more poor families; without their unpaid work the poverty experienced by families would be far worse. But the responsibility of women for unpaid work is also a key factor *causing* women's poverty. Women, because they bear the responsibility for domestic work and childcare, are more restricted in the labour market than men. Thus they are less likely to be employed at all, less likely to have full-time jobs, they work in a more restricted range of jobs and are more likely to be low-paid (Lonsdale, 1992). Their opportunities for the sort of jobs that provide the best protection against poverty – permanent, full-time, full-year employment – are heavily restricted by their responsibilities for caring, not only for children but also for other dependent family members (McLaughlin, 1991). The sexual division of labour, which assigns the primary role of women to be in the home and that of men to be in the labour market, is the main reason why women have less command over resources than men and thus why they are at a greater risk of poverty.

The consequences of this sexual division of labour are wide-ranging and inter-linked and have the effect of creating a vicious circle of disadvantage for women. Because women have primary responsibility for the home they are not able to put paid work first; because they do not put their jobs first they are not the breadwinners and so they have less of a claim on the family income; because they are not breadwin-ners it is not important if they earn low pay and there is no need for the state to pay them benefits if they lose their jobs. Financial dependency, and the fact that so many women do not have an adequate income of their own, is not seen as a policy issue. In fact quite the reverse is the case. For example, the Wages Councils, which set minimum wages for low-paid workers in certain industries, were abolished in 1994 (agriculture excepted). Women are particularly likely to be working in jobs that were covered by Wages Councils agreements but the government argued that women did not need this protection because most women live with a partner who is the primary wage earner. According to this perspective women are thus not considered as poor even when they earn poverty-level wages. This ignores the increasing number of women who live without a male partner, as lone mothers or as single women. It also ignores the fact that such low wages inevitably mean financial dependency on others.

Thus an assumption of the financial dependency of women on men continues to structure women's access to resources in the labour market, the family and – as the next section discusses – the social security system.

Women and social security benefits: the limits to equal treatment

Writing in the war years, when women were playing a key part in both the armed forces and the civilian labour market, Beveridge was nevertheless clear that the appropriate division of labour between the sexes meant that women should be at home and men out at work. He sums this up when discussing the treatment of married women in his proposed national insurance scheme: 'The attitude of the housewife to gainful employment outside the home is not and should not be the same as the single woman – she has other duties' (Beveridge, 1942: para. 114). Under the Beveridge plan, which laid the foundations for the current social security system, the needs of married women were to be covered in two ways: firstly, by means of provisions intended to support their role as mothers (maternity benefits, children's allowances, marriage grant); and secondly, by entitlement to support through their husbands' national insurance contributions (as dependants if their husbands were claiming benefits; as widows; as separated or divorced women.)[2] According to Beveridge, marriage and motherhood should be women's careers and their financial support should be either through the wages earned by their husbands, or through his membership of the national insurance scheme. There was, Beveridge argued, no need for married women to have benefit entitlements in their own right; instead their rights would be derived from their husbands. To reinforce this further, the 'married women's option' also effectively excluded those married women who *were* employed outside the home. These women could have contributed in their own right and thus earned their own benefits but were encouraged not to do so under the 'married women's option'. This allowed employed married women to opt out of the scheme and, since there was nothing to be gained financially by being a member, most did opt out (Pascall, 1986; Lister, 1992).

This discrimination against married women continued for thirty years until, in 1977, the married women's option was abolished. Married women are now eligible to claim national insurance benefits on the same basis as men. They may also be the claimant of income support which, up until 1983, had to be claimed by the man in a couple. Other examples of discrimination against women – the exclusion of married women from the invalid care allowance, the 'household duties test' imposed on disabled women but not on disabled men and the fact that women could not claim benefits for their husbands as dependants – have also been removed from the system. Thus direct discrimination against married women has been largely eliminated from the social security system. The immediate stimulus for much of this change came from Europe and, in particular, the 1979 Directive on Equal Treatment in Social Security. These European Directives are binding on member states although the actual means of implementation are left to each country to determine. This 'milestone in the treatment of women in the social security system' (Lister, 1992: 26) removed direct discrimination in provisions for women of working age (it does not apply, however, to occupational schemes, nor to survivors' benefits, nor to pensions) and thus, when implemented, gave women the same benefit entitlements as men.

As with the Equal Pay Act, however, the focus of this approach is very much on procedural equality – on ensuring that men and women in the same circumstances are treated in the same way, with no discrimination, direct or indirect, allowed on the grounds of sex. This equality in treatment, however, does little to change the underlying inequality between men and women. As Pascall (1986: 208) puts it: 'In an equal world this would be an incontestable advance for women. In a world where women work for low pay and often part time . . . it will not bring equal security.' In practice women continue to have more restricted access to social security benefits than men for three main reasons.

Firstly, the national insurance scheme is tied to male, rather than female, patterns of employment. In general, women are lower-paid than men with many more women working part-time. This means that a large number of women – about 2.25 million – are excluded altogether from the national insurance scheme because they earn below the minimum needed for entitlement (Lister, 1992). If they lose their jobs, therefore, they have no entitlement to national insurance benefits. Nor are they entitled to statutory maternity pay. For those women who are making national insurance contributions, their lower pay means that they take longer than men to earn entitlement and, in the case of earnings-related pensions, ultimately receive lower amounts of money. Women also have more interrupted employment histories than men, primarily because of breaks in employment to care for children or other dependants. These breaks reduce entitlement although the 'home responsibilities credits', which safeguard basic pension entitlement during such periods of caring, do provide women with some protection. However, women still have to have twenty years of contributions or credits to qualify for a full pension (Walker, 1992). Women pensioners are among the poorest members of our society and only about a third of the current 6.5 million women pensioners have qualified for a pension in their own right (DSS, 1993). Furthermore, because many women are excluded from national insurance benefits in their own right then many continue to rely upon their husbands' contributions. This leaves them very vulnerable in the case of divorce when they stand to lose these derived pension rights (Joshi and Davies, 1991).

Secondly, the national insurance scheme does not adequately recognise, and compensate, the circumstances that led to gaps in employment for women but not for men. The most obvious example is maternity. Statutory maternity pay is currently paid to those women who earn above the national insurance threshold and who have worked for the same employer for at least 26 weeks. A higher rate is paid to those who have worked for the same employer for at least 16 hours per week for two years or at least eight hours per week for five years. Compared with other European countries, these conditions are restrictive and the level of maternity pay received is low. A survey in 1988 found that about 69 per cent of employed pregnant women received statutory maternity pay, 42 per cent at the higher level. Rather fewer – 60 per cent – qualified for the right to reinstatement (McRae, 1991). Under pressure again from Europe, the government has recently announced that the lower rate of maternity pay will be increased and some women will become eligible for the higher rates after six months' employment. It is estimated that about 285,000 women per year will benefit from these changes.

Other forms of caring – for children or for other dependants – are not part of the national insurance scheme (except, as noted above, through home responsibilities credits). Child benefit is paid to mothers on behalf of their children but has been frozen throughout much of the 1980s. The main benefit available to carers is the invalid care allowance, a non-contributory benefit which is paid to someone providing care for a recipient of one of the disablement benefits. But invalid care allowance is set at a low rate and cannot be received on top of other benefits such as income support. It thus neither compensates for lost earnings nor provides an adequate income on which to live (McLaughlin, 1991). Unpaid caring work, one of the main reasons why women have different employment patterns from men, is thus recognised only very partially in the social security system.

Thirdly, the direction of recent policy, in which means-tested rather than national insurance benefits play a more important role and where family and private support are stressed, further erodes independent entitlements for women. National insurance benefits have, in practice, become less and less important in recent years as more and more people find themselves outside the scope of these benefits. This is partly because of the growth of both long-term unemployment and more casualised patterns of work, with men particularly affected by the former and women by the latter. It is also the result of deliberate government policy in which the better 'targeting' of benefits has been, and is, a key policy objective. Thus income support has become the main benefit received by those not in work and in 1992 there were 5 million people claiming this benefit and a total of 8 million people – one in seven of the population – living in families receiving it (DSS, 1993). Income support is a means-tested benefit, paid for the family as a whole, on the basis of total family income. Thus women who are married to employed husbands will usually be unable to claim income support, whatever their personal incomes and needs. In addition the rules make it financially unrewarding for women married to unemployed men to carry on in employment themselves and many women in this situation give up work and so lose their own source of income (Millar, 1989). Couples 'living together as man and wife' are treated in the same way as married couples and for many lone mothers this has led to a particular scrutiny of their circumstances with the benefit withdrawn from those deemed to be living with a male partner whether, in reality, he is financially support-ing her or not. The concepts of breadwinner men and financially dependent women remain strong in the rules surrounding means-tested benefits.

They also remain very strong in the child support legislation, introduced in 1991 and implemented – to severe criticism – from 1993. The Child Support Act aims to get more absent fathers to pay more money in child support than has usually been the case hitherto. However, even if this can be achieved, most lone mothers will not benefit financially because all child support is deducted pound for pound from income support.

The objective of decreasing public dependency on benefits by increasing private dependency through child support will not help the majority of lone mothers to improve their incomes but will leave them worse off in terms of autonomy and independence (Clarke *et al.*, 1993; Millar, 1996). Other moves to encourage more self-support through, for example, private and occupational pensions also hold heavy risks for women (Groves, 1992). Only 39 per cent of employed women are members of occupational pension schemes compared with 58 per cent of men and about 1.9 million women have private pensions compared with 3.4 million men (DSS, 1993). Again, women's low-paid and discontinuous employment puts them at a disadvantage, and their poverty during working life is thus carried with them into old age.

    Finally, for those who must rely upon them, benefit rates are low and, it has been argued, are insufficient to keep those in receipt out of poverty. The study by Kempson *et al.* (1994), discussed above, is one in a long line of studies describing the struggle of those living on income support to make ends meet. The work of the Family Budget Unit, who have costed the price of a 'modest-but-adequate budget' and a 'low-cost budget', also demonstrates the failure of income support to meet needs. The modest-but-adequate budget is far beyond the means of families on income support and the benefit rates could only meet 74 per cent of the low-cost budget for a couple with two children and 77 per cent for a lone parent with two children (Bradshaw, 1993).

Social security policies for women

The current social security system provides the main source of income for many women but it fails to provide adequacy and security. What reforms to social security would best meet the needs of women? One option would be for benefits to be 'individualised', that is paid to individuals on the basis of their individual entitlement and intended to meet their needs alone. This would mean that each person would have to earn their own benefit entitlement and there would be no assumptions made about financial dependency among couples. As Lister (1992) points out, there had been some interest in the idea of individualised benefits within the European Commission, not least because of concerns about the loss of derived pension rights among divorced women. Income support (and other means-tested benefits) could either be paid individually (that is, asseessed as now but the payment split between the couple) or both assessed and paid individually (which might involve taking account of any income transfers to the claimant from his/her partner). Splitting payments might simply reinforce ideas of his and her money and so actually reduce intra-family transfers. A fully independent scheme would be costly, would involve even more means-testing and could lead to more women dropping out of employment (Esam and Berthoud, 1991; Duncan *et al.*, 1994).

    An alternative is to try and move away from means-testing and to seek both to restore the importance of national insutrance benefits and to make them fit more closely the needs of women. The latter is particularly important because there are obvious dangers for women in simply abolishing derived rights and expecting all women to be able to earn their own benefit entitlements. As discussed above, women's caring responsibilities do limit their participation in employment and this needs to be taken into account. One possibility would be to drop, or substantially amend, the contribution conditions so that more women – and especially part-time workers – are brought into the national insurance net. In addition, new benefits could be introduced to cover the specific needs of women, for example a parental care allowance to be paid to those who stay at home to care for children. Such benefits, however, raise a difficult dilemma: would they 'lock women further into their caring role in the "private" sphere of the family and out of the labour market and the "public" sphere more generally' (Lister, 1992: 68)? Benefits for caring might improve the independent access of women to social security benefits but at a cost of reducing their chances of gaining an independent income through employment.

Parker (1993) argues that much more fundamental reform is needed, in the form of a 'citizen's income', which would provide all adults, and children, with an income in their own right. She argues that this would have many advantages for women, including greater autonomy and choice about working and living arrangements, more recognition of the value of unpaid work, and more financial independence for women within families. Basic income schemes are, however, inevitably expensive as well as sitting somewhat uneasily with the value placed upon employment as the main source of income in our society.

Social security benefits offer both opportunities and constraints. On the one hand, benefits can free people from dependence on other sources of income. They act as an alternative to wages so that those who have entitlements to benefits can survive outside the labour market. As Esping-Andersen (1990: 37) puts it, benefits can 'decommodify'; they can allow people to 'uphold a satisfactory standard of living independently of market participation' and that possibility can give people greater freedom, for example, to refuse low wages or poor working conditions. Similarly, as Lister (1994) and McLaughlin and Glendinning (1994) have pointed out, benefits can free people from financial dependency on other family members ('defamilialise') and, in particular, can free women from dependence upon men by allowing women an income in their own right. On the other hand, however, social security benefits are not given freely and the conditions attached to benefits also act as a control or constraint upon choices. Benefits operate to enforce labour discipline, for example by excluding those with poor work records from receipt and by keeping benefit levels down in order to encourage claimants into low-paid work. Similarly, social security benefits can be structured to support particular family structures and gender roles. The Beveridge model clearly supported one view of the way families should be organised. However, changes in the family and employment lives of both women and men have made this approach seem increasingly out of date. Constructing a system that more closely reflects contemporary patterns of life is the challenge facing the system now and essential if the rising level of poverty is to be reversed.

Notes

1. Some studies are based on household measures (i.e. all those who live together) and some on family (i.e. usually defined as single people with or without dependent children and couples with or without dependent children). Household-based measures produce lower poverty estimates than family-based measures (see Roll, 1992, for further discussion). However, from the point of view of the argument here, similar criticisms apply and so household and family are used interchangeably in the following discussion.
2. Not all the measures proposed by Beveridge were actually introduced. The marriage grant never appeared, nor did his proposed separation benefit, for women who divorced or separated (see Millar, 1996, for further discussion).

5   *Women and housing*

Roberta Woods

Women find it harder to gain access to housing which is allocated by ability to pay rather than by housing need. Changes to housing policies since 1979 have made it increasingly difficult to gain access to public sector housing and there is greater emphasis on finding housing in the private sector – especially through owner occupation. Such a trend produces increasing disadvantage for women. (Muir and Ross, 1993: 1)

This chapter seeks to document the way in which the direction of national housing policy since 1980 has created difficulties for female-headed households with regard to accessing good-quality affordable housing. Much of the broader women and housing literature addresses the debate between gender roles and the importance of the built environment in the construction of those roles (Little *et al.*, 1988; Roberts, 1991; R. Gilroy, 1993). Consideration in the literature is also given to the question of whether a home has a particular meaning for women as many women spend considerable periods of time there. Darke (1994) has explored the contradictory relationship that women may have with the home – the safe haven versus the site of exploitation. Finally, the importance of security and safety in housing design and creating women friendly spaces has also been addressed (McDowell, 1983; Kelly, 1986; Ahrentzen and Franck, 1989). This chapter, however, contributes to the literature (see Brailey, 1985; Sexty, 1990; Muir and Ross, 1993) that has focused on problems with allocations policies and the structural disadvantages that place women in a weak situation with regard to the provision of housing.

The above statement from Muir and Ross sums up in a nutshell the effect of 1980s housing policies on women. In general terms the focus of central government policy has been aimed at reducing the resources that are available to social rented housing for repair and maintenance and new building and has concentrated on private forms of housing provision, most notably through encouraging expansion in owner occupation. Specific policy measures such as the 'Right to Buy' sections of the Housing Act 1980, which gave local authority tenants the right to purchase their property, have been accompanied by the rehearsal of strong ideological arguments against direct state involvement in the provision of housing. This led to further legislation in the form of the Housing Act 1988 and the Local Government and Housing Act 1989, which sought to undermine the role of local authorities as direct providers of housing and instead encouraged them to adopt an enabling role of securing housing for tenants from a range of agencies including private landlords and housing associations. Housing has therefore been included in the attack on collective means of meeting social needs that have been common to a number of areas of social provision since 1979. As this chapter shows, women rely heavily on the state sector to provide them with housing and the effects of the attack on this sector for women are considered below. In sum, it can be noted that the promotion of a privatised system of housing provision has meant that women are less likely to be owner occupiers, are over-represented in local authority housing (also referred to as council housing); and when they do access owner occupation it is to poorer-quality housing. The literature has shown that with lower earnings women find it harder to access good-quality accommodation in a housing system that is market-based (Brion, 1987; Morris and Winn, 1990; Sexty, 1990).

Women and council housing

Data on women's access to council housing are not easy to come by. Local authorities are under no obligation to provide information about family type with regard to lettings and while many local authorities do routinely collect these data, many do not. Nevertheless there is now considerable evidence that female-headed households are over-represented in local authority housing. On the face of it this may seem to contradict previous literature which has documented in detail the difficulty that women face with regard to accessing council housing. This is not necessarily the case as women generally access council housing because they fall into a vulnerable category with regard to homeless persons legislation; that is, they have children, are elderly or are pregnant. Single women are unlikely to gain access to local authority housing unless they are able to place themselves in one of the vulnerable groups covered by part 3 of the 1985 Housing Act.

There are, however, three other issues to be considered in addition to access to local authority housing: those of quality of accommodation, location and affordability. Preliminary results from a survey of allocations in twenty local authorities suggest that female-headed households are more likely than other family types to be housed in maisonettes or flats.[1] Similarly, such households are more likely to be found clustered in the more run-down estates and they are less likely than other household types to be allocated properties in areas with low scores on a deprivation index. Despite problems with regard to location and quality of stock, this tenure remains very important for female-headed households.

Prescott-Clarke *et al.* (1994) found that among applicants for local authority housing lone parents had the lowest incomes. Reasons given in this survey for wanting council housing are particularly relevant to women: 70 per cent of applicants with children said that affordability was the main reason for being on a waiting list. Other reasons given for wishing to access council accommodation included many older people wanting sheltered accommodation, a majority of whom were women.

These authors also found that 80 per cent of lone parents considered themselves to be in very or fairly urgent housing need. This compared with 73 per cent for two-person households with children, 31 per cent of single pensioners and 28 per cent of pensioner couples. Single parents were found to spend the least time on the waiting list. Lone parents spent a median of 1.1 years on the waiting list compared to 1.4 years for couples with children and 1.7 years for couples with no children. This is a likely reflection of their degree of housing need. As we explore later, many single parents will access local authority accommodation through the homeless persons legislation.

As shown in Table 5.1, in England, of those households renting from the local council in 1988, 44 per cent were couples, 17 per cent were single parents, 5 per cent were multi-person households, 12 per cent were one-person male households and 23 per cent were one-person female households (Department of the Environment (DoE), 1993). This pattern had changed by 1991, but only slightly. The number of couple households reduced to 41 per cent whilst the number of lone-parent households rose to 18 per cent and female single households to 24 per cent. Table 5.1 shows a similar pattern for housing associations. The private rented sector, however, has only 12 per cent of its stock let to lone parents in both 1988 and 1992. Private renting is more important to single female households, with the respective figures for 1988 and 1991 being 22 and 21 per cent for furnished accommodation and 17 and 15 per cent for unfurnished accommodation.

Table 5.2 shows the importance of each type of tenure for various household types. Whilst the figure for single males buying with a mortgage is 43 per cent, the corresponding figure for females in 1988 was only 22 per cent. In 1991, the two groups had moved slightly closer together with 39 per cent of single men and 25 per cent of single women buying a property with a mortgage.

Widowed men and women show a similar tenure pattern in both 1988 and 1991; but the picture shows large differences in tenure with regard to divorced and separated men and women. In 1988, 39 per cent of divorced or separated men were buying a property with a mortgage, whilst in 1991 the corresponding figure was 44 per cent. For women, the percentage figure was 31 per cent in 1988 and 33 per cent in 1991.

Table 5.1 Households in England in 1988 and 1991: sex and marital status of head of household

Tenure	Couple	Lone parent		All lone parents	Other multi-person	One male person	One female person
		With depend-ants	Without depend-ants				
1988							
Rented from council	44	12	5	17	5	12	23
Rented from housing association	32	14	3	17	6	13	32
Rented privately unfurnished	48	4	3	7	8	14	22
Rented privately furnished	15	4	1	5	32	31	17
All rented privately	39	4	3	7	15	19	21
1991							
Rented from council	41	12	6	18	3	13	24
Rented from housing association	37	10	3	13	3	15	32
Rented privately unfurnished	50	5	2	7	5	16	21
Rented privately furnished	28	3	2	5	26	26	15
All rented privately	43	5	2	7	12	19	19

Source: Adapted from Department of the Environment (1993: Table 2.1)

Forty-two per cent of divorced or separated women occupied a council house, with a further 5 per cent renting from a housing association. In 1991, 39 per cent of divorced or separated women rented from the council and 6 per cent from a housing association. The corresponding figures for divorced and separated men are much lower, with 29 per cent of them renting from the council and 3 per cent renting from a housing association in 1988. In 1991, 25 per cent of divorced or separated men rented from a local authority and 3 per cent from a housing association. The figures clearly indicate the relative importance of the two main tenures (owner occupation and local authority renting) for male and female households. Women are over-represented in rented housing and under-represented in owner occupation, with the exception of widowed households.

The heavy reliance that women face on accessing council housing means that changes imposed on this sector by central government since 1980 have had particular effects on women. Many of the changes relate to the Right to Buy legislation (a provision that enabled tenants to purchase their council house introduced by the 1980 Housing Act). Evidence in this chapter and elsewhere (Munro and Smith, 1989;

Table 5.2 Sex and marital status of head of household by tenure: households in England 1988 and 1991

Sex and marital status of head of household	Tenure								
	Owner-occupied				Privately rented				
	Owned outright	With mortgage	All	Council rented	Housing associ- ation	Unfur- nished	Fur- nished	All	Total
1988									
Male									
Married	25	51	76	17	1	5	1	6	100
Cohabiting	–	–	–	–	–	–	–	–	100
Single	13	43	55	18	3	9	14	24	100
Widowed	45	8	53	34	3	9	1	10	100
Divorced or separated	14	39	53	29	3	10	6	15	100
All male	24	48	72	18	2	6	2	8	100
Female									
Married	–	–	–	–	–	–	–	–	100
Cohabiting	–	–	–	–	–	–	–	–	100
Single	21	22	42	32	7	9	9	19	100
Widowed	46	5	50	37	4	8	–	9	100
Divorced or separated	14	31	44	42	5	7	2	8	100
All female	32	15	47	37	5	8	3	11	100
Total	26	40	66	23	2	7	3	9	100
1991									
Male									
Married	25	54	79	13	2	5	1	6	100
Cohabiting	4	59	63	17	3	10	8	17	100
Single	14	39	53	18	4	10	16	26	100
Widowed	46	9	55	33	5	7	1	7	100
Divorced or separated	12	44	56	25	3	10	6	15	100
All male	23	51	74	15	2	6	3	9	100
Female									
Married	–	–	–	–	–	–	–	–	100
Cohabiting	–	–	–	–	–	–	–	–	100
Single	19	25	44	31	6	9	10	19	100
Widowed	46	6	52	35	5	7	1	8	100
Divorced or separated	13	33	46	39	6	7	2	9	100
All female	31	18	49	35	6	8	3	11	100
Total	25	43	68	20	3	6	3	9	100

Source: Department of the Environment (1993: Table 2.1a)

Sexty, 1990; Muir and Ross, 1993) shows that women are less likely than men to be able to purchase a property. Right to Buy sales, many of which have been of the best housing stock, have thus reduced the quality and quantity of council housing that is available for those who must rely upon it to meet their housing need.

Table 5.3 documents the sales of public sector housing stock between 1981 and 1991. The table shows that over 1,300,000 homes have been taken out of the local authority sector. This may not necessarily have presented a problem for people needing to access local authority housing had the homes been replaced. Table 5.4, however, shows that this has not been the case. New building in the local authority

Table 5.3 Right to Buy sales: Great Britain

Year	All sales	Local authority sales
1981	82,404	79,430
1982	202,396	196,430
1983	144,289	138,511
1984	104,769	100,149
1985	95,865	92,230
1986	93,782	89,250
1987	108,033	103,309
1988	167,609	160,568
1989	190,166	181,367
1990	132,450	126,210
1991	77,104	173,458
Total	1,399,065	1,340,912

Source: Adapted from Department of the Environment (1993: Table 9.7)

Table 5.4 Permanent dwellings started: Great Britain

Year	Private sector	Housing associations	Local authorities[1]
1981	117,367	11,567	23,787
1982	140,790	18,272	32,769
1983	172,405	14,255	32,376
1984	158,335	12,651	26,159
1985	165,682	12,453	20,839
1986	180,006	12,997	19,185
1987	196,814	12,905	18,849
1988	221,404	14,422	15,347
1989	170,122	15,808	14,060
1990	135,252	18,671	7,671
1991	134,920	21,588	3,713

Note: [1] includes Scottish homes
Source: Adapted from Department of the Environment (1992: Table 6.1)

sector has virtually ceased. During the 1980s the government stated that it wished housing associations to become the main providers of social rented housing, but the figures show that new building by housing associations has not kept pace with the depletion of the local authority stock. Table 5.4 shows clearly the emphasis that has been placed on the private sector, primarily building for owner occupation, since 1981. An important question, then, is how do female-headed households fare with regard to accessing owner occupation?

Barriers to accessing owner occupation

Watson (1988) highlighted the discriminatory policies of building societies as a contributory factor in the difficulty women faced in entering owner occupation. Such direct discrimination is now considered rare. Instead, indirect discrimination is thought to be more important (Glithero, 1986). A consideration of the lower earnings of women is central to this issue. Women are simply not able to afford owner occupation and, when they do, they must commit more of their earnings to do so (Nationwide Anglia Building Society, 1989, 1994). Muir and Ross (1993) state that given women's average wages, and house prices for flats in the lowest decile of house prices in London, only 15 per cent of women could afford to buy (Muir and Ross, 1993: 27). Similarly only 19 per cent can afford the price of a bedsit. The reasons are obvious and are based on women's employment patterns and their levels of pay. Female levels of pay both in terms of gross weekly incomes and hourly rates fall behind those of men.

Table 5.5 shows that women earn significantly less than men. The earnings of women are further depressed when one considers the number of women working part-time. Data from the General Household Survey show that, of women who have dependent children, 42 per cent of married women and 24 per cent of lone mothers work part-time whilst 21 per cent of married women and 15 per cent of lone parents work full-time.

Similarly, information from the Child Poverty Action Group highlights the comparatively high number of single parents, most of whom are female, who rely on state

Table 5.5 Average gross weekly earnings of males and females in full-time employment: Great Britain

	Average weekly earnings (£)
Males non-manual (full-time)	400.4
Males manual (full-time)	268.3
Female non-manual (full-time)	256.5
Female manual (full-time)	170.1

Source: *New Earnings Survey*, (1992)

Roberta Woods

Table 5.6 Social security claimants by sex: Great Britain

Benefit	Men (%)	Women (%)
Invalidity benefit	76	24
Retirement pension	35	65
Unemployment benefit	68	32
Attendance allowance	37	63
Mobility allowance	52	48
Severe disability allowance	40	60
Family credit	1	99
Income support	43	57

Source: Adapted from R. Lister, *Women's Economic Dependency and Social Security*, Equal Opportunities Commission, 1992, quoted in Oppenheim (1993; 98)

Table 5.7 Tenure type by household

Tenure	Type of household						
	Couple	Lone parent			Other multi-person	One male person	One female person
		With depend-ants	Without depend-ants	All lone parents			
1988							
Owned outright	58	2	4	5	4	9	23
Buying with mortgage	77	4	2	5	7	6	5
All owners	70	3	3	5	6	7	12
1991							
Owned outright	58	1	4	5	4	9	24
Buying with mortgage	79	4	2	6	3	8	5
All owners	71	3	3	6	3	8	12

Source: Adapted from Department of the Environment (1993: Table 2.3)

benefits. More women than men can be seen to rely on the main means-tested benefits of income support (Table 5.6). The way in which this low income translates into buying properties is shown in Table 5.7.

Table 5.7 shows that of those households who are buying a property with a mortgage 77 per cent were couple households in 1988 with this figure rising to 79 per cent in 1991. Lone-parent households buying with a mortgage were 5 per cent in 1988 and 6 per cent in 1991. For those who own their property outright 58 per cent were couple households in both 1988 and 1991. Single-male households comprised 9 per cent of those who owned outright in 1988 with the corresponding figure for female single households being 23 per cent. The respective comparators for 1991 were 9 and 24 per cent. Further data from the DoE (1992) show that the relatively high number of females in this category is accounted for by a large number of widows in this group.

Table 5.8 Housing affordability

		ibution (%)		
		)00–,999	£20,000+	Total %
R UNIVERSITY OF WOLVERHAMPTON		5	4	100
R Harrison Learning Centre		2	3	101
P₁ ITEMS RETURNED:		3	8	100
P₁		1	11	100
R Title: welfare of Europe's children : are EU		5	6	99
O member states converging?		2	33	100
O ID: 7623969601		2	13	98

Sc Total items: 1
07/10/2008 13:40

e 12.1)

Thank you for using Self Service.
Please keep your receipt.

Overdue books are fined at 40p per day for
1 week loans, 10p per day for long loans.

given in Table 5.8. This table
per cent have annual incomes
hose renting from a housing
with a mortgage fall into this
only 7 per cent of those with
uthority or a housing associa-
with a mortgage fall into this
al authority is £7,500, from a
age is £18,700. This informa-
ition is firmly linked to house-

Private renting

The government plans[2] to introduce changes to the homeless persons legislation so that the right of those who are considered to be homeless to permanent accommodation will be replaced by a duty to find them temporary housing for twelve months. The DoE has indicated that it wishes the private rented sector to have a greater role in providing housing for single parents and other vulnerable groups who are currently housed as a priority under the homeless persons provisions of the 1985 Housing Act. Yet there is much evidence to demonstrate that this sector is particularly unsuited to homeless people (Blake, 1994a). Most of the criticisms of the private rented sector concentrate on five areas: insecurity of lettings, availability, cost, possible harassment from landlords and lack of support for those with particular care/social needs.

Insecurity of lettings, availability and cost

The 1988 Housing Act contained within it measures that the government hoped would revitalise the private rented sector. All new lettings were to become 'assured' or 'assured shorthold' tenancies. Assured tenancies brought with them fewer rights of security for tenants; shorthold tenancies can be terminated after a six-month period; assured tenancies gave increased rights to landlords to enable them to seek repossession of their property. Additionally the system of fair rents which had covered rents in the private sector was replaced by market rents. It was hoped that by giving landlords greater return on their money the sector would become more attractive to potential investors. Much of the private rented stock is out of reach to people on low incomes. Cheaper properties are likely to be of poor quality. Figures from the latest House Condition Survey show that this tenure has a high rate of disrepair. Availability is also an issue: the size of this tenure has been in sharp decline since the Second Wold War and it currently accounts for only 7.4 per cent of the housing stock (see Table 5.9). It is clear that this tenure cannot replace council housing as the main provider of housing for homeless people (Blake, 1994b). A very high degree of investment would be necessary to enable it to accommodate large numbers of homeless families even for the temporary one-year period that is proposed.

Harassment from landlords

There is some evidence that women occupying private sector lets are at some risk of harassment from their landlords (Watson and Austerberry, 1986; Miller, 1990; Thornton, 1990). Thornton (1990: 26) reports that:

> The GLC study of 1983–1984 found that 12% of women living alone in privately rented accommodation had suffered serious molestation. And in a survey of women's safety in 1984, 1% of all rapes reported had been committed by the victim's landlord.

Table 5.9 Stock of dwellings by tenure 1981–91: Great Britain

Stock	Owner occupation	Rented privately	Rented from housing association	Rented from local authority or New Town Corporation (NTC)
1981	11,701 (55.8)	2,353 (11.2)	453 (2.2)	6,447 (30.8)
1986	13,811 (62.7)	1,892 (8.6)	551 (2.5)	5,776 (26.2)
1991	15,601 (67.7)	1,704 (7.4)	724 (3.1)	5,017 (21.8)

Source: Adapted from Department of the Environment (1992: Table 9.3)

Similarly Miller (1990: 27) states that twice as many women as men suffer harassment and poor living conditions in the private rented sector. She notes that this is particularly the case with regard to Black women, lesbians and elderly women who are living alone. Such evidence suggests that the government's suggestions to use this sector to house homeless people on a temporary (one-year) basis in the future are particularly inappropriate for women, some of whom will be vulnerable to abuse or harassment from landlords.

Lack of support for care/social needs

Striking differences between the social rented and private rented sectors are the welfare functions that are undertaken as part of routine housing management. In particular, local authorities are in a position to develop close working relationships with social services departments to give support to particular tenants. This may be part of an individual's community care plan or part of a wider community development strategy aimed at providing resources to local communities and housing estates. A question to be asked is what experience do private landlords have in dealing with the welfare functions of housing management?

> Doubts also linger about most landlords' abilities to cope with the added responsibility that can come with housing people on lower incomes. Families on benefit often need welfare support and advice and those in work do not. Council and housing association managers have the training and experience to cope with these demands. Can landlords renting out just one property really do the same job? (Blake, 1994b: 27)

The support that is given to tenants with particular social needs is also at risk from the compulsory competitive tendering of housing management. If local authorities lose the contracts to manage their stock it is debateable whether the new landlords will carry out the welfare and community development functions currently undertaken by many local authority landlords.

This section has documented the difficulty that women face in accessing good quality accommodation across a range of tenures. The chapter turns next to the impact of demographic trends and relationship breakdown on women's need for housing and to the particular needs of various groups of women.

Demographic trends

Demographic trends, such as the creation of new households on family break-up or the growing number of female single households as women outlive men, are relevant to a consideration of meeting housing needs. The General Household Survey shows that in 1992 females accounted for 53 per cent of the population aged between 65 and 69, 56 per cent of the population aged between 70 and 74, and 62 per cent of those over 75. Fifty-nine per cent of women aged over 75 were living alone compared to 30 per cent of men in this age group. The growing number of single-parent households and single-person households has contributed to an overall reduction in the average household size. Our concern here is that it creates a need for more housing units.

Women's economically disadvantaged position means that they are often not able to continue in the family home as owner occupiers (Symon, 1990). If enough equity is available they may be able to move down market to a cheaper property. Information that is available shows that female-headed households access the cheapest and poorest-quality owner-occupied housing (Nationwide Anglia Building Society, 1989).

Relationship breakdown

The rehousing of female-headed households on relationship breakdown is currently the subject of much controversy, as is the housing of single parents generally. Recent research by Bull (1993) has shown that a majority of single parents occupied local authority housing but she also notes that after relationship breakdown there are a large number of women who are without a permanent home of their own and who stay with family and friends. Whilst this is a common theme across tenures, it is particularly pronounced with regard to owner occupiers. Bull (1993) found, however, that long-term changes of tenure are not common; 91 per cent of local authority tenants and 77 per cent of owner occupiers stayed in the same tenure following relationship breakdown. Where shifts of tenure did take place they were generally from owner-occupied to local authority housing. Of those who had moved tenure 63 per cent felt that their new accommodation was much the same in terms of quality; only a minority considered their new accommodation to be better:

> Net tenure movements following relationship breakdown were from owner occupation and private renting into local authority housing. The share of those in local authority housing increased from 43 per cent to 54 per cent after relationship breakdown. The percentage in owner occupation decreased by 5 per cent. The share of the total accounted for by housing associations remained stable at 4 per cent. (Bull, 1993: 14)

Stability of tenure should not imply that people have stability of housing. Evidence from a DoE survey (Bull, 1993) shows that the majority of tenants who had remained in the social rented sector had moved from their original tenancy. The report notes that moves out of owner occupation were the most frequent, with about half of owner occupiers moving to local authority housing following relationship breakdown. They also note, in line with McCarthy and Simpson (1991), that those who remain in the owner-occupied sector are likely to be custodial parents, most of whom are women.

The housing options that women have available to them upon relationship break-down rely heavily on the policies of their local authority. To date, much evidence has documented the variation in policies across local authorities to the treatment of women in these circumstances (Brailey, 1985; Logan, 1986; Institute of Housing, 1987). Policies of the local authority are sometimes related to the consideration of family law with regard to who gets custody of the children and the family home. Policies that will vary relate to how women with or without children are treated if they are fleeing domestic violence, how women who already have a tenancy are dealt with, and the quality and quantity of advice on their housing options. What is beyond dispute is that relationship breakdown is one of the main reasons that women give for applying as homeless to local authorities for accommodation.

A diversity of needs

There is a tendency when thinking about women's housing needs to group women together as if their collective needs were not differentiated in any way. This is, of course, not the case. Darke (1987, 1989) and Morris and Winn (1990) have pointed to the need to consider the housing needs of different groups of women. The next section will look at the housing needs of young women, elderly women, Black women and lesbians.

Young women

Young women who do not wish to remain in the family home or find that they are unable to stay there because of their personal circumstances have a very limited range of housing options available to them. Homeless young women have no right to accommodation under homelessness legislation. They may be able to access local authority housing if the local authority chooses to place them in one of the vulnerable categories covered by the legislation. A young woman may be placed in this category if she is able to show that she is at risk of physical or sexual abuse in the family home; however, many young women are unable or unwilling to disclose this information to housing agencies. Some local authorities do consider all sixteen- and seventeen-year-olds to be generally 'at risk' but this is by no means common practice.

Young women may also be unable to secure accommodation in the private rented sector. If a young person is able to afford accommodation in the private rented sector it is likely that it will be of poor quality and will probably be a house in multiple occupation (HMO). For some considerable time the government has been under pressure to tighten the inspection laws relating to HMOs to make them safer living environments. Regulations introduced under the Local Government and Housing Act 1989 went some way towards forcing landlords to be responsible managers of their properties. There remains a problem in ensuring that local authorities have the necessary resources to carry out their inspection and enforcement tasks. As the section on private renting above states, young women may be at risk of abuse or harassment in this tenure.

In addition many private lets require rent in advance or deposits before a tenancy can be granted. Such payments are not available through the social security system and the low income of young people makes it difficult for them to save money for downpayments. Some housing agencies are now providing assistance for young people with rent deposits but it is as yet not widespread practice.

There are also a number of schemes throughout the country that provide supported accommodation or support services to young people to help them establish themselves in a tenancy. These can include providing support workers, advice and liaison with relevant agencies or furnished or part-furnished accommodation. Again the availability of such support varies greatly across local authorities.

Changes in social security regulations in 1986, enacted in 1988, have meant that young people, especially those under twenty-five, receive less money. Reliance on the social fund for meeting or attempting to meet one-off needs rather than obtaining a grant can mean that it is difficult for young people who rely on social security to obtain money for essential furniture. Indeed most sixteen- and seventeen-year-olds are prevented from getting income support; instead they must attend a YTS scheme.

It is, then, not surprising that young women find it difficult to access owner occupation. Table 5.10 shows that for females under thirty the most relevant tenancy is local authority accommodation, although owner occupation and private renting are also important. The use of housing association accommodation is growing but still only accounts for 7 per cent of accommodation for this group. Comparable figures for young men show much greater reliance on owner occupation, with council housing being much less important and private rented accommodation of lesser relevance also.

Table 5.10 Sex of household by tenure for under-thirties

Sex and age of household	Tenure (%)								Total %
	Owner-occupied			Council	Housing association	Privately rented			
	Owned outright	With mortgage	All			Unfurnished	Furnished	All	
1988									
Male under 30	4	59	63	16	2	8	11	19	100
Female under 30	2	24	26	42	7	10	16	26	100
1991									
Male under 30	2	60	62	14	2	10	12	22	100
Female under 30	1	23	24	41	7	11	16	27	100

Source: Adapted from Department of the Environment (1993: Table 2.2a)

Elderly women

It would be quite wrong to suggest that the housing experience of elderly women is uniform. To a large extent the housing situation of elderly women reflects their housing history. Some elderly women will be able to remain in the family home with a home owned outright or will trade down or sideways to more suitable accommodation; others will stay in their rented tenancy in the private or public sector or move to sheltered accommodation, again in the public or private sector. Figures from the DoE (1992) show that 46 per cent of women aged over sixty-five owned their home outright. A further 36 per cent were in council accommodation, 6 per cent were in housing association homes and 12 per cent were in the private rented sector.

Sykes (1994) shows that elderly women owner occupiers are concentrated in the older housing stock with a poor record on their state of repair. It is often then difficult for them to maintain a good quality of housing whilst remaining in the family home. Similarly, as they get frailer it may be difficult for them to get the necessary aids and adaptations to the property to cope with their growing disability (Brotchie and Hills, 1991: 46). Community care is of some assistance here, as are some of the schemes run by housing associations such as Anchor's 'Staying Put' scheme, which enables elderly people to stay in their homes by providing a range of support services (see Smith, 1989).

Black women

Recent statistics from the General Household Survey show the tenure profile for ethnic minorities to be as shown in Table 5.11. The heavy reliance of some ethnic minority groups on owner occupation does not necessarily mean that they are in good-quality accommodation. Many Asian families may enter owner occupation because there is no alternative available to them:

> Asian households have been caught in a 'catch 22' situation. Excluded from council housing through the effects of residence qualifications and forced into poor standard owner occupied housing, the self-reliance of Asian families is now being used as the reason for their subsequent exclusion from the local authority sector. (Amin with Oppenheim, 1992: 22)

Other ethnic minorities – most notably Black Caribbeans – do rely more heavily upon the social rented sector. This is, of course, not always an option as immigration laws can require that people who are allowed to enter this country do so on the condition that they do not have recourse to public funds. Residential qualifications may also prevent Black people from gaining access to council housing.

Black women have particular problems. Rao (1990) notes the particular problems faced by Black women trying to access council accommodation. They had to wait

Table 5.11 Housing tenure by ethnic group of head of household

Tenure	White (%)	Indian (%)	Pakistani/ Bangla- deshi (%)	Black Caribbean (%)	Remain- ing groups (%)	All ethnic minority groups (%)	Total (%)
Owner-occupied, owned outright	25	15	12	8	10	11	25
Owner-occupied, with mortgage	41	65	54	38	41	48	41
Rented with job or business	2	2	2	1	3	2	2
Rented from local authority/new town or from housing association or co-operative	26	10	22	47	32	29	26
Rented privately unfurnished	4	3	3	3	4	3	4
Rented privately furnished	2	5	6	3	11	7	2
Base = 100%	28,267	310	160	304	406	1,180	29,447

Source: OPCS (1992: Table 2.19)

longer than White women, were offered poorer properties and were not offered transfers at the same rate as White women; in fact they hardly featured in transfer procedures at all. Black women also find it hard to access owner occupation. Oppenheim (1993: 118) provides some evidence to show that, like other groups of women, Black women suffer from low pay.

Across all sectors Black women are subject to racial harassment. In Rao's study (1990) 32 per cent of women said that they had been racially abused; the same number had experienced racial assaults and 23 per cent had suffered some form of damage to their property. Her findings reinforce those of two reports from the Commission for Racial Equality (CRE) that showed Black women to be at a disadvantage across all housing tenures (CRE, 1989a, 1989b). She also uncovered evidence of non-reporting of attacks as Black people had little belief that the police, local authorities or private landlords would intervene on their behalf. A number of local authorities have developed policies specifically aimed at trying to prevent racist attacks on tenants. These include taking court action against perpetrators of racial abuse and violence by seeking repossession of their property. There is also a growing trend of using injunctions to prevent persons from carrying out racist attacks. All too often, however, a 'solution' to the problem is obtained by moving the people who are being attacked or abused to another property.

Lesbians

A number of studies have referred to the invisibility of the housing needs of lesbians (Dibblin, 1988; Egerton, 1990). Lesbian couples may find it hard to get a local authority tenancy. Additionally young lesbians may find hostel accommodation unsuitable or inappropriate to their needs. At the outset lesbians may find it hard to articulate their needs, as housing providers may be unsympathetic to them. When a relationship breaks down lesbians can be particularly vulnerable as local authorities will not recognise the homelessness of one of the parties involved. This means that the two sectors that may most appeal to lesbians are owner occupation or private renting. As a consequence of this they may face higher rents or greater housing costs through owner occupation.

Housing policy – the good news?

As this chapter shows, trends in housing policy since 1980 have marginalised women's housing needs and limited the choices that are available for them. It is, however, possible to argue that some of the measures introduced did allow the prospect of addressing some aspects of women's housing needs, albeit indirectly. Provisions contained in the 1986 Housing and Planning Act and the 1988 Housing Act (for a full description of the acts see Walentowicz, 1990; Ward 1990) to enable local authorities to transfer their stock to another landlord or to enable tenants to choose a new landlord pushed providers of social housing towards greater involvement of tenants in the management of their stock. This has important implications for women. Much of the participation was to involve liaising with tenants' associations and many of the members of such associations are women. At the same time these proposals and those to establish housing action trusts stimulated activity in the tenants' movement largely through opposition to these proposals. It seemed, towards the end of the decade, that the government had inadvertently ushered in a new breed of social landlord that was willing to speak to and meet with tenants, consider their views and in some cases share management with them through tenant management boards. Alas, it would appear that the government commitment to tenant participation was based on the assumption that, if given the choice, local authority tenants would choose another landlord. When they consistently rejected choosing another landlord, voluntary transfer and Housing Action Trusts, tenant participation must not have appeared such a good idea.

If 'tenant participation' were the buzz words of the late 1980s, 'compulsory competitive tendering' are those of the 1990s. With its zeal for tenant participation dampened, the government repealed a section of the 1986 Act to ensure that tenants would not be able to have a veto over landlords who may compete for a local authority housing management contract. The wishes of tenants to remain with the local authority managers will be ignored. Instead local authority contracts will be awarded on the basis of price and a range of management tasks and performance indicators that must be adhered to. But there is another factor to be considered here. Many of the problems facing people today in public housing estates, such as high levels of crime, unemployment and a need for improvements in the social and physical environment, require an input from a range of agencies in and beyond the local authority sector. Local authorities working with local community groups are often in the best position to co-ordinate the multi-agency approach that is necessary to tackle the problems identified above. Women are often at the forefront of the campaigns to get improvements and better resources for their areas. There is a very real fear that if the local authority housing management contracts are lost to other landlords then so will the opportunity be lost to create multi-agency strategies to improve housing estates and the quality of life for people living there.

Tenant participation varies by degree amongst local authorities and housing associations. The London Borough of Lewisham and York City Council pioneered involving tenants directly in quality assessment. Others are carrying out or piloting a range of joint management initiatives with the aim of developing closer links with tenants and negating the image of local authorities being aloof bureaucratic landlords. Whilst such initiatives remain there is at least the possibility that some women will have their views about the state of repair of their dwellings, the quality of their environment and the needs of their community taken into account. Direct face-to-face contact with local housing managers is a key feature of tenant participation. Involving tenants is still an important aspect of the work of many local authorities and housing associations and a number of them have continued to develop participatory mechanisms for tenants despite a change in government rhetoric. However, it remains to be seen whether tenant participation will stay a central feature of housing management should contracts go outside current social landlords. If this is the case, then an opportunity for many tenants to influence the delivery of housing services in their area will be lost.

The second development which may be considered to have helped women is the encouragement during the 1980s of the provision of low-cost housing for sale and a range of part-buy, part-rent schemes. Unfortunately there are limited data available on the gender breakdown of who is benefiting from low-cost home ownership. Data from Cousins *et al.*, quoted in Gilroy (1994), are moderately encouraging. They suggest that people purchasing under such schemes had lower incomes than the median income of single people and lone parents. They also state that 14 per cent of shared ownership purchasers were formerly in owner occupation and that 27 per cent of this group were divorced or separated. This information might suggest that women who were owner occupiers are able to take advantage of such schemes upon relationship breakdown. The lower incomes required to enter shared ownership are also likely to help women.

Conclusions

Evidence suggests that policies pursued since 1980 to promote home ownership at the expense of support to other tenures do not help women. Choices for those who do not aspire to, or cannot attain the 'dream' of, owning their own home have not been adequately resourced and the residualisation of council housing has not helped those people with low incomes, many of whom are women, who must depend upon it.

Notes

1. The project is funded by the ESRC and involves an examination of the allocations policies and practice of twenty local authorities in England and Wales. The grant holder is the author of this chapter.
2. In January 1994 the government issued a consultation paper entitled *Access to Local Authority and Housing Association Tenancies*. This was followed by a press statement in July 1994 which indicated that key sections of the consultation paper regarding the removal of the right to permanent accommodation for homeless people would be sought.

6   *Women and educational reform*

Rosemary Deem

Introduction

This chapter explores some of the consequences of recent educational reforms and restructuring of state education for women in the United Kingdom. In so doing no unity is assumed across the United Kingdom, which consists of four distinct countries, Wales, Scotland, Northern Ireland and England, each with their own particular features and characteristics, although there are some shared elements of education reform in all four. Nor is it assumed that women as a category are homogeneous, since there are probably almost as many differences among women in the United Kingdom as there are similarities. Age, ethnic group membership, social class and ablebodiedness or disability are just some of the characteristics which make it necessary to examine carefully any tendency to generalise to all women; all of these are crucial dimensions of educational processes and experiences. Nevertheless there are sufficient patterns in common in both the structuring and the content of reforms, and in relation to women's experiences, for the exercise to be worth while. In particular, it is possible to examine the extent to which gendered processes and discourses are apparent in widespread changes to education which might appear at first glance to be gender-neutral. First I will examine the patterns of recent UK education reforms, asking whether, and if so how, they have taken gender into account, before going on to explore some of the possible consequences for women in relation to four key themes: diversity, sex education, the involvement of lay people in school governance and the effects of educational reform on women staff in schools.

Although the article focuses primarily on educational reform, not on feminist theories, it is worth while saying something at this point about theoretical perspectives. As Middleton and Yates have noted, there has been a significant shift in the dominant theoretical frameworks used to analyse women's education over the past three decades (Middleton, 1993; Yates, 1993). The liberal, socialist and radical feminist analyses which were so influential in the late 1970s and early 1980s examined changes in relation to equal access to educational opportunities, looked at strategies emphasising the relationship between gender, class and the labour market, highlighted classroom interaction, power relations and language, and encouraged the development of equal opportunities and anti-sexist policies in educational institutions. These theories have given way to Black feminist critiques of the White-centric nature of previous approaches and greater emphasis on post-structuralist and postmodernist feminist theories. The theories of the 1970s and early 1980s put a great deal of emphasis on the category of woman as distinct from man, using gender in a relatively unproblematised manner. Attention was also paid to apparently universal concepts (for example, patriarchy, relations of production and ideology) which sought to explain the determinations of gender stereotypes and relations. In addition there was emphasis on developing generally applicable change strategies for rendering gender relations in education less unequal. By contrast, postmodernist and post-structuralist ideas pay much more attention to differences among women, as well as differences between women and men, reject universal theories and political strategies for change, substitute the term 'discourse' for ideology and place a lot of emphasis on examining, in particular local contexts, the contradictory discourses within which girls and women are positioned, arguing that this leads to a range of identities, rather than just those of femininity.

As Yates and Middleton have observed, the influences of these more recent theories have not been confined to academic feminism but can be seen to have influenced educational policies in a number of countries, including the United Kingdom, Australia and New Zealand (Middleton, 1993; Yates, 1993). New developments in feminist theory cannot and should not be ignored, especially since they are both motivated by and have influenced political events. However, it is important that we do not allow the current fashion for focusing on difference and identity, to distract our attention from the possibility that the economic, the political and the cultural have a more systematic influence on inequalities than might be supposed from an analysis which concentrates only on the politics of the differential identities of women. As Steedman (1994) notes, such an individual approach whereby 'the hidden injuries of class, the hurts of racism . . . ways of thinking and feeling that are actually about enmity between communities of people – are elided with the fascinating individual differences from each other that people may feel they have' may actually prevent us from recognising that some differences are neither random nor the product of 'choice' (Steedman, 1994: 62). So whilst I pay attention in the rest of the chapter to the recognition of diversity and multiple identities amongst women, I also

examine the extent to which recent education reforms are gendered and the consequences of these reforms for considerable numbers of women in the United
Kingdom.

Educational reform and restructuring

Educational reform is a phenomenon not confined to the late twentieth century or to the
United Kingdom. Furthermore, the motivations and intentions behind educational
reform policies are many and varied. Whilst economic reasons have often been to the
fore, desires to reduce inequality, variously defined, have also been features of reform
programmes. In addition, however, as social policy analysts have pointed out, policy
processes are almost inevitably subject to unintended consequences (Ham and Hill,
1984). Thus, even if the reduction of inequality is an explicit intention of educational
restructuring, as was the case with the move from selective to comprehensive secondary
schooling in England and Wales in the mid-1960s, we cannot assume that this will
necessarily be the outcome. Conversely, reforms with no intention of addressing inequality may turn out in retrospect to have done so. Reforms and restructuring of
education during the 1980s and 1990s in a number of western democracies appear to
have shared some of the same characteristics, including greater parental and student
choices of establishment, the development of quasi-markets for publicly funded education, the devolution of financial and management responsibilities to the school or college
level, emphasis on educational and moral standards, and more involvement of lay
people in the administration of educational institutions. These similarities are clearly of
interest to the student of social policy, not least because they suggest that some measure
of 'policy borrowing' may be occurring across different countries (Halpin and Troyna,
1994). However, as Halpin and Troyna note, such borrowing is not necessarily related
so much to the supposed 'success' of particular policies, as to the attempt to legitimise
certain kinds of policy developments and directions. Hence 'policy borrowing' may be
more likely when different education systems have similar characteristics, as well as
shared political ideologies and discourses.

Keeping a comparative and historical perspective is as important in the study of
social policy as in other areas of the social sciences but it is also crucial that we do not
assume *a priori* equivalences in the shaping and consequences of what may appear to
be similar changes (Deem, 1994b). Thus, as Brown (1994) and Jarman (1994) have
noted, although there are a number of seemingly indistinguishable characteristics of
recent education reform to be found in Northern Ireland, Scotland and England, for
example a desire to involve the consumer of education more fully in the process of
schooling, there are also features distinctive to each of those countries and the
response to the reforms has also varied. It is in addition salutary to remember that
some education reforms, including those in the United Kingdom to which this
chapter refers, may be partly triggered by economic crisis rather than economic
growth (Ginsburg *et al.*, 1990). Concomitantly, we might expect to find that reforms

in recessions do not have the same kinds of outcomes for gender and other aspects of social inequality as do those which take place in periods of economic prosperity.

England and Wales

This section traces some of the major characteristics of educational reform in England and Wales between the mid-1980s and the mid-1990s and enquires whether any of these explicitly set out to tackle gender or other aspects of inequality. It is not entirely satisfactory, though necessary here because of space limitations, to treat England and Wales together, despite their common education reform legislation, as there are significant differences between the two, politically, economically and culturally. These differences include the importance of Welsh as a first language and key part of the National Curriculum and testing in many Welsh schools, and the different administration of education in the Principality, through the Welsh Office rather than the Department for Education. In respect of both school reforms and higher education there have been signs of different policies and/or differing responses to them in Wales as compared to England. These actual and potential differences between England and Wales should be borne in mind throughout this section.

During the 1970s, ideas about the adoption of core curricula in schools in the interests of gender equality were much emphasised as a way forward, partly to overcome the apparent tendencies of girls in England and Wales to specialise in humanities and social science subjects, and boys to concentrate on maths and sciences (Byrne, 1978; Deem, 1978). By the 1980s these suggestions had been superseded by demands that teachers, educational institutions and local education authorities (LEAs) should try to establish policies tackling sexism at a more general level than option choice (Arnot, 1985; Whyte *et al.*, 1985; Arnot and Weiner, 1987). In the 1990s, concerns have turned to examining the consequences of educational reform and the need for more far-reaching equal-opportunities policies to meet the differential requirements of girls and women (Arnot and Weiler, 1993; Siraj-Blatchford, 1993; Weiner, 1994). One view, dominant at the moment, is that reforms aimed at improving things for girls and women in education have not necessarily been successful, sometimes leading to greater regulation and surveillance in education than previously, and that more general educational reforms have not really taken gender issues seriously enough (Arnot and Weiler, 1993; Middleton, 1993; Yates, 1993). In England and Wales the 1980s educational reforms included a considerable measure of centralised curriculum and assessment control in schools, leading to National Curricula for each country and national assessment systems for five- to sixteen-year-olds involving benchmark tests at the ages of seven, eleven, fourteen and sixteen across a range of subjects. Although these changes were not intended to tackle gender issues, there was initially some optimism that they might at least facilitate a greater degree of fairness. However, as commentators have shown, concerns about gender, ethnicity and other kinds of cultural bias have not so far made much impact on curriculum and assessment policies (Arnot and Weiler, 1993; David, 1993; Gipps and Murphy, 1994; Weiner, 1994). In any case the reforms have been difficult to evaluate fully. Between the 1988 Education Reform Act and 1994, the nature of the curriculum and assessment had already undergone quite radical changes, with further educational legislation, including the 1992 Schools Act and the 1993 Education Act, as well the recommendations of the Dearing Report, which attempted to deal with complaints about an overcrowded curriculum and a greatly increased teacher workload (Dearing, 1994). Nevertheless, there was some initial optimism that reforms to curricula and testing would help reduce gender differences across different subjects. Furthermore, some groups saw plans to keep parents more informed about their children's progress by publication of test scores as a potentially important development, especially for Black parents (Blair, 1993).

Other aspects of educational restructuring have affected those who teach rather than what they teach, including conditions of service, teacher training and school inspection. Since 1987, the working conditions of teachers, and more recently those of lecturers in the formerly LEA-controlled further- and higher-education sectors, have been more tightly controlled and regulated by the state than previously, as have their salaries. In further-education establishments, this has taken the form of attempts to introduce more flexibility into the hours taught (including evening and weekend work), a lengthening of the working week and reductions in holiday entitlement. Such changes might be expected to have a particular effect on women teachers who are also mothers or who have other responsibilities for the care of dependants, since flexible alternative care arrangements can be very difficult to arrange (David, 1993).

Since the early 1990s there have also been endeavours to shift more teacher training from higher education into schools and to increase the practical rather than theoretical aspects of that training. This might be seen not to have had any particular impact on women except that rising numbers of women are entering teaching; in 1990/1 56 per cent of teachers in the United Kingdom as a whole were women, compared with 52 per cent in 1980/1. Although in the 1990s more women are entering higher education than previously, with a 76 per cent increase in their participation between 1980/1 and 1990/1 (Government Statistical Services, 1993), it is still much more likely that women will enter teacher training. Hence endeavours to sever some or all of the links between teacher education and the mainstream of higher-education provision might be expected to affect more women than men. Such a divide not only provides a form of segregating post-school education but one in which it is particularly difficult to monitor the existence or effectiveness of the kinds of equal-opportunities policies advocated by feminist and ethnic minority critics of teacher education (Flintoff, 1993; Siraj-Blatchford, 1993). Ironically, the attempts through Project 2000 to make nursing an all-graduate profession have moved in the other direction, locating much more of nurse training in higher-education institutions than was previously the case.

UK state schools have long been subject to systems of nationally organised inspection. However, in England and Wales the inspection system for state schools has undergone a thoroughgoing set of changes since 1992, with the *de facto* privatisation of inspection systems and the introduction of lay as well as professional inspectors under the auspices of the Office for Standards in Education (OFSTED). Although there were never large numbers of either Her Majesty's or LEA inspectors who were women, there are now very few women indeed in the newly privatised service; they formed only 2 per cent of registered inspectors in 1994. Although the 1992 Schools Act and the inspection criteria laid down for schools showed some awareness of equal-opportunities issues, including 'race' as well as gender, with inspectors asked to examine equal opportunities in achievement and learning, school policies and the implementation of those policies, we cannot assume that all this necessarily takes place. Thus Harris found in fifteen randomly selected reports of the first tranche of published school inspection reports in 1993–4, that only five made any reference to equal opportunities at all, each quite limited in scope (Harris, 1994). In higher and further education, mechanisms enabling the monitoring of quality assurance systems, educational standards, teaching, and, in higher education only, research, have been introduced. Here the representation of women on audit teams and assessment panels is better than for OFSTED but tends to reflect the lower number of women in senior positions in universities. For example, by 1994 only 5 per cent of professors were women (in 1991 it was 3 per cent), despite the increase in the numbers of women obtaining chairs as the former polytechnics became universities, and historical subject divisions between the sexes persist in higher education. Thus, for instance, there are far more women involved in the assessment of social policy teaching than there are in physics.

Changes to teaching and its surveillance systems have been accompanied by measures giving greater autonomy and local control, including financial delegation to schools and colleges, often exercised under the joint responsibility of heads or principals in conjunction with lay people. The latter are not themselves expected to possess significant amounts of educational expertise (Deem, 1994c). However, research on the impact of these changes on both governors and school staff (Broadbent and Laughlin, 1993; Broadbent *et al.*, 1993) has suggested that women do not always play as full a policy-shaping role in local management as they might (Deem, 1990).

Decentralisation of the running of schools, sometimes called site-based or local management (LMS), has also been accompanied by the total removal of local education authorities from any oversight of grant-maintained status (GMS) schools. In GMS schools, after a parental ballot in favour of the change, schools are funded directly from the Funding Agency for Schools rather than by an LEA. GMS schools have proved notably more popular in England than in Wales. Sixth-form and further-education colleges, former polytechnics and colleges of higher education have also been given the status of independent corporations rather than operating under LEA control, though again the patterning and pace of these changes were different in Wales. In the case of those state schools remaining under LEA control, there has been a huge reduction in the powers of those LEAs. Consequently, democratically elected local bodies, once responsible for the planning, resourcing and strategic development of education in an entire area, have been replaced with bodies which are at best semi-democratic, as with school governing bodies where only parent and teacher governors are elected, or entirely unelected, as in the case of the governing bodies of post-compulsory educational institutions. This development is one of many which support the view that unaccountable quangos are replacing democratically elected bodies in the exercise and monitoring of public policy (Stewart *et al.*, 1992; Cohen and Weir, 1994; Hackett and Pyke, 1994). Governing bodies of state-funded educational institutions, whether elected or not, now have quite demanding responsibilities, including finance, strategic planning and the hiring and firing of staff. In recently completed research on school governing bodies, I and two other researchers found that governing body sub-committees dealing with finance and personnel issues were often male-dominated (Deem 1990, 1994c). A national study of governing bodies of further education colleges found that 92 per cent of chairpersons and 80 per cent of members of those governing bodies were male (NATFHE, 1993). Hence the voices of mothers, women teachers, business women and female community members may not always be heard in the making of key decisions in governing bodies.

Another feature of the English and Welsh reforms has been the development of 'quasi-markets' in education (Le Grand and Bartlett, 1993). Under the provisions of the latter, publicly funded schools and colleges are expected to compete for students who, together with their parents, are enabled to exercise some degree of choice over the educational establishment attended. The National Curriculum and national assessment are seen as providing both a consistent system of schooling and indicators of individual and school performance which can be used by parents in making decisions about which school they want their children to attend. A considerable amount of research has been done or is in progress about parental choice of mainstream schools but, as David (1993) notes, this research does not seem to take into account gender relations in respect of the relative roles of mothers and fathers. Nor does it explore in any detail whether the processes of school choice are the same for girls as for boys (David, 1993). Yet, as Riddell (1992) has shown, mothers often foster ambitions for their daughters which are specifically shaped by their experience of gendered schooling, employment and household life. Nor has there been any research which looks at the ways in which women and girls choose further- or higher-education institutions, although there is some excellent qualitative small-scale research work documenting the experience of mature women students in higher education (Edwards, 1993).

In both school and post-compulsory sectors, the move to quasi-markets has been underpinned by a system of funding based largely on student numbers. In higher education this aspect of entrepreneurial activity proved too attractive and in 1993 severe limits were placed by the government on further expansion. It is too soon to know whether the pressures on other educational institutions to try to recruit as many students as they can cram in will have any significant gender effects. However, the ways in which educational markets appear to work suggest that social class, ethnicity and the attainment levels of the young people concerned are important factors shaping the extent to which parents and students can exercise any meaningful choice of school (David, 1993; Bowe *et al.*, 1994).

National Curriculum, national assessment, quality assurance mechanisms, changes in working conditions of educational workers, site-based management, quasi-market formation and student/parental choice represent attempts to alter both the infrastructure of public education and the culture of the institutions which provide it, encouraging a more business-like ethos, which emphasis on entrepreneurial activity, budgets, performance indicators and targets. This cultural shift is sometimes referred to as 'enterprise culture' (Keat and Abercrombie, 1991) but is undoubtedly unevenly distributed across institutions. It is assumed by the instigators of educational reform that fostering an 'enterprise culture' will result in educational institutions which are more responsive to the needs of its consumers, and higher educational standards. It is too soon to know much about the possible connections between enterprise culture and gender relations in educational settings; however, given the continued dominance of the business world by men, it seems possible that enterprise culture may conflict with some of the more educationally orientated, caring and humanistic cultures which characterise some educational organisations, especially those where women are in the majority (Acker, 1992a).

Cross-UK differences in education reform: Scotland and Northern Ireland

I now turn to a consideration of the Scottish and Northern Ireland reforms, examining points of similarity and difference and asking whether these reforms also have any particular consequences for women. The educational systems which exist in each country in the United Kingdom are somewhat different and so too are the political and social contexts of those systems. In England and Wales there is a majority of secular schools but there are also denominational schools which receive funding from the state. All primary and most secondary schools take children of all attainment levels but there are still selective secondary schools in some areas. GMS schools (which are wholly state-funded) and city technology colleges (CTCs), which are part-state and part-privately funded, can select pupils according to attainment level, although not all do so. In Scotland, although there is also a mix of secular and religious denominational schools, the majority of state-funded secondary and primary educational establishments admit a comprehensive ability range of pupils without use of selection tests. Provision for self-governing schools (comparable to GMS schools) exists but by mid-1994 only one school had chosen this route. In 1994 there were as yet no technology academies (the Scottish equivalent of CTCs). Lay involvement in schools is in the form of School Boards but the Boards contain only parents, co-opted members and teachers, not headteachers, who may only attend, or local authority representatives. Scottish Board members also have a much narrower range of responsibilities than is the case in England and Wales. The Scottish regional educational authorities (EAs) retain many of their powers, unlike their English and Welsh counterparts, but they are being broken up into smaller units which may affect the level of services and resourcing they can provide. Reforms to further and higher education have followed similar lines to those in England and Wales but Scotland's Higher

Education Funding Council has taken a different stance on a number of issues, including the methodology for assessing teaching quality. Interestingly, the Welsh Higher Education Funding Council is also now taking a different line on this from the English Council.

Curriculum changes for five- to fourteen-year-olds have taken place in Scottish schools but there is no equivalent of the National Curriculum and what does exist is less prescriptive, with less emphasis on the separation of subject areas. In Scotland there is a long-standing tradition of students taking a broad range of subjects right up to school-leaving age and higher-education entry; no such tradition exists in England and Wales. Thus the concerns raised by feminists about option choice in schools have never been such a live issue in Scotland. Indeed, whilst in England until very recently girls only outperformed boys at GCSE level (taken usually by sixteen-year-olds), in Scotland girls have consistently done better than boys not only in Standard Grade exams but also in Higher Grade exams, the equivalent of A-levels. The 1989 Scotland Education Reform Act attempted to introduce national testing to schools in somewhat similar ways to England but met considerable resistance from both parents and teachers, with the protests much greater in extent than in England and Wales.

Although devolved school management (DSM) is being introduced into Scotland, it is not based on a single centrally determined formula as it is in England/Wales and this may permit more sensitivity to local inequalities than has been possible in England or Wales. It is still too early to tell how gender relations will be affected by this system of local management but it is possible that, as in England, women will end up in the servicing roles and men in the policy-making roles.

Parental choice in Scotland was developed to a greater extent under the 1981 Act than the rather vague expression of parental preference made possible by the 1980 Act in England. However, parental choice of any kind is limited in the many rural areas of Scotland and there is evidence of a much higher degree of parental satisfaction with local schools than is the case in England (Adler *et al.*, 1989; Brown, 1994). As in England, there do not appear to have been any studies of how the gender of parents or students affects the choice process.

Scotland also differs from England in a number of other crucial respects, including national politics, culture and the economy. Scotland returned a high anti-Tory vote in the 1992 General Election (this is also a pattern found in Wales). Many of the educational reforms that have been attempted in England are regarded with disdain because they are perceived as evidence of 'Englishness'. As far as the overall situation of women in Scotland is concerned, the percentage of adult women in employment is not dissimilar to that of England (51.2 per cent in Scotland as against 53.1 per cent in England), although unemployment rates are generally lower than in England (Central Statistical Services, 1993). However all the official UK unemployment figures mask female unemployment because of the ways in which women who are married and/or mothers are discouraged from registering as unemployed.

Northern Ireland presents a rather different picture again as far as reform is concerned. Some of the reforms have been along parallel lines to those in England and Wales, particularly with regard to the National Curriculum and assessment, although the fine detail of curriculum and testing differ in some important respects from those in England and Wales. Devolved management is also run on quite similar lines to those operating in England and Wales. There are no democratically elected education authorities in Northern Ireland; instead, state-funded schools are run by Education and Library Boards (ELBs), which are quangos without any revenue-raising powers, and education funding is via the Northern Ireland government Department of Education (DENI). The membership of the ELBs is overwhelmingly male. The organisation of schooling at secondary level is very different from the rest of the United Kingdom, with non-selective state schools, a tiny number of controlled grammar schools, Catholic maintained schools, voluntary Protestant and Catholic grammar schools and a few integrated (Protestant and Catholic) GMS schools. No other kind of GMS schools are permitted under the Northern Ireland legislation. Governing bodies of schools have an extensive range of responsibilities comparable to those in England and Wales, with a much higher predominance of male governors (McKeown, 1994) than is the case in England (Keys and Fernandes, 1990).

Politically, the contest of the civil conflict in the province and the existence of the sectarian divide between Protestants and Catholics, even if the current signs of peace look more hopeful, cannot help but influence the ethos and culture of Northern Ireland education. There is a high level of unemployment in Northern Ireland as compared to the rest of the United Kingdom, especially amongst Catholics and for those in employment there is a smaller percentage of adult women who are in employment as compared with the remainder of the United Kingdom. Yet in other respects Northern Ireland is more favoured, with a lower cost and higher standard of living and less crime than the rest of the United Kingdom. As in Scotland, there appears to be a relatively high amount of satisfaction with school education in the province (Jarman, 1994). As far as women are concerned, a basic framework of anti-sex-discrimination exists as in the rest of the United Kingdom, although there is a separate Equal Opportunities Commission for Northern Ireland. However, many of the major concerns with equal opportunities in the province have focused around the sectarian divide rather than around gender, and as a consequence it is the question of equal treatment for Catholics alongside Protestants that has often been the centre of equal-opportunities policies, with gender and other social divisions taking more of a back seat.

Gendered education reform policies

Having explored in some detail both the extent to which educational reform is gendered and the variations as well as similarities across the United Kingdom in relation to educational restructuring, I want now to explore four themes and concerns relevant to women in education which arise out of aspects of policies developed in some of the recent UK reforms. As David (1993) has noted, much educational research has failed to take into account the gendering of policies but, where possible, I draw on research which has taken this into account. Where there is no relevant published research, I suggest what kind of research agenda is needed. Partly for reasons of space, and also because of my own research expertise, I have chosen themes which are related to compulsory schooling, though several of them are equally applicable to other sectors of education.

From equality to diversity?

One of the features of contemporary education reform in the United Kingdom has been the focus not on equal opportunities but on diversity. This rather ambiguous term can appear congruent with the emphasis placed on identity and difference by recent developments in feminist and other social theory, and thus suggest a coalescence between the ideas of social scientists and politicians. However, any assumption about shared meanings could be misleading. In 1992 a government White Paper entitled *Choice and Diversity: A new framework for schools* appeared in England, setting out various options for further educational reform. The main definition of diversity seemed to be in relation to different types of schools (LEA, voluntary and GMS and City Technology Colleges), rather than in respect of pupils. There was almost no mention of equal opportunities let alone gender in the paper, and the section on spiritual and moral development talked about the need to pay 'Proper regard . . . to the nation's Christian heritage and traditions.' In a country where there are many different religious faiths as well as secular traditions this does not sound much like recognition of diversity!

In countries like New Zealand, the recognition of diversity has enabled the development of new policies on the education of ethnic minority groups, though some NZ writers indicate that Maoris still find themselves very dissatisfied with what is offered in mainstream education (Smith, 1993). However, although paying attention to diversity may have positive consequences for some groups, especially students and parents from ethnic minority groups, in recognising that they have needs, interests and concerns which are different from those of ethnic majority groups, this emphasis does not necessarily also have positive outcomes for issues relating to gender. It can result in gender relations being ignored altogether, particularly by governments, teachers and schools who do not regard gender as a legitimate concern of educational establishments. We do not yet know what effects the attempts to produce diversity in school provision have had on gendered patterns of achievement and learning but a system not set up to address those issues directly is not well placed to respond.[1] Furthermore, whilst it is possible to see how diversity can be used in constructive ways in teaching and learning, celebrating difference rather than erasing it or rendering it invisible, if we extend this to the policy level it can become more problematic for two reasons. Firstly, it may mask gendered patterns of achievement and learning which are neither random nor accidental and thus mean that insufficient resources are devoted to solving problems which are about collectivities rather than individuals. Secondly, it is an impossible task to collect national or international data which are cognisant of all or even most individual differences; we are still struggling in the United Kingdom to get basic statistical data broken down by gender and by ethnic group, let alone something much more complex. Yet without those data it is impossible to know what is happening either at a national or at an international level and there is no sound basis for future planning.

Sex education

Issues raised by educational reform in relation to sex education illustrate the kinds of problems raised when insufficient attention is paid to gender relations in policy formulation. Sex education is a very controversial area of the school curriculum in many countries and it is frequently linked to other ideas and values about religion, heterosexuality, 'family life' and morality. Many teachers feel uncomfortable about teaching sex education either because it preys on their own sexual identity and insecurities about sexuality or because they are aware that what they teach is capable of being interpreted and misinterpreted in many different ways by parents (Shucksmith *et al.*, 1994). Sometimes what is taught can become rather detached from the actual experiences of young people or is inappropriate to the audience. Thus Measor found adolescent girls studied by her were embarrassed by having to watch birth films in mixed groups (Measor, 1989). Issues like menstruation may also be insensitively handled (Prendergast, 1989).

Despite the existence of sex education in many UK schools, it often seems to have little impact on those for whom it is provided. Recent extensive studies of sexual behaviour in young people show that girls are often very ignorant about how their bodies work, know little about contraception and have only slight knowledge of male/ female power struggles over sex in heterosexual relationships. AIDS is seen as something that only happens to people living in certain areas, homosexuals or those who engage in casual sex (Thomson and Scott 1990a, 1990b; Holland *et al.*, 1992). The ignorance of the role of gender power relations in sex also seems to extend to those who work in schools. As Holly has shown, pregnant schoolgirls can be treated extremely badly by schools and when they resume their education they may do so in a special unit or with a private tutor rather than returning to school (Holly, 1989).

In England and Wales, changes to school sex education have been part of the recent agenda for educational reform. The 1986 Education Act gave school governors and headteachers the responsibility of deciding whether or not sex education should take place in school and, if it did, for determining its content. Under the same act, LEAs, governing bodies and headteachers became responsible for ensuring that where sex education was given, pupils were encouraged to have due regard to moral considerations and the value of family life (Section 46). In the research which Kevin Behony, Sue Hemmings, Suzanne New and I did on English school governing bodies from 1988 to 1992, we observed little or no direct discussion about sex education in meetings of governors. Where it was discussed, a policy was often adopted with little debate. Under the 1993 Education Act, the situation has been altered. In primary schools governors may still decide whether sex education is to be taught or not and may determine what is to be taught. In secondary schools sex education is now compulsory but parents have the right to withdraw children from it; parents of primary children have also been given the same right. Details about AIDS, HIV, sexually transmitted diseases and human sexual behaviour are no longer permitted as part of the National Curriculum and can only be taught in sex or personal and social education, for which little time is left. During 1994 the English Department for Education attempted to draw up guidelines for sex education for schools, and during this time a number of controversies involving sex education arose in the media. All of these focused on whether sex education should concentrate on 'facts' or on relationships and, if on the latter, what kinds of relationships should be emphasised. Many of those participating in the debates seem to have been influenced by religion and other moral and ethical principles but rarely by any awareness of how strongly gender and sexual identity affect both sexual behaviour in young people and other power relations between the sexes. The findings of recent research on young people's sexuality and sex education and the importance of gender to both of these have scarcely influenced what happens in schools. The research evidence suggests that single-sex classes for sex education are essential, yet very few mixed schools in the United Kingdom appear to provide these. Those who are not employed directly by schools may be more likely to offer such provision (Shucksmith *et al.*, 1994). Almost the only issue where gender is taken at all seriously is in relation to teenage pregnancy and, as Holly's (1989) work shows, that is often in a negative way. Sex education is indeed an interesting example of the practice of the normalisation of gendered power relations in such a way that it is not even questioned by the majority of those involved in sex education. However organisations like the Sex Education Forum demonstrate that it is possible to have a public impact on the debates around sex education whilst also being well informed about gender, sexual behaviour and sexuality (Sex Education Forum, 1993). There are considerable implications for girls and women of the current state regulation of sex education, especially in relation to their struggle for sexual identity and relationships, irrespective of sexual orientation, in which they exercise power and control. Sex education is both intensely private yet regulated by the state. Here diversity and choice seem to matter less than particular definitions of morality, which themselves seem singularly inappropriate in a pluralist society.

Lay involvement in school governance

Here I draw on recent research carried out by a team of four people: myself, Kevin Brehony, Sue Hemmings and Suzanne Heath. We tracked all the meetings and activities of ten contrasting primary- and secondary-school governing bodies in two different English LEAs for the four years immediately after school governance in England and Wales was significantly reformed by the 1986 (no. 2) Education Act and the 1988 Education Reform Act (Deem and Brehony, 1993). As well as keeping extensive fieldnotes, we also interviewed key actors, used questionnaires and analysed documentation used by the ten governing bodies. Previous research on governors had not addressed gender issues and it was not seen to be of any significance. Our research has demonstrated that this is not the case. Amongst the issues we uncovered were the gendering of the organisational structures and cultures of governing bodies, gendered interactions (and silences) in governing body meetings, and a failure on behalf of most governing bodies we studied to address matters of gender and other equal-opportunities concerns in schools.

In examining the maze of governing body sub-committees established from 1989, when such sub-committees became common practice in English and Welsh schools (Baginsky *et al.*, 1991), we found that female and male governors were not distributed either randomly or equally to different committees but that key resource-handling groups dealing with the concerns of finance, staffing and building were dominated by men. Those sub-committees more central to teaching and learning tended to have mixed or female-dominated membership (Deem, 1990, 1994c). Formal governing body meetings need to be clerked by someone who is not themselves a governor, in order to produce a written record of the meeting and the decisions taken. In all but one of our research sites this role was carried out by women, whether school or LEA employees, who were generally poorly paid for their services and frequently treated as though they were inferior to the governors themselves. One female clerk whose school had already exhausted the money set aside for her pay that financial year because of long and extra meetings, offered her a bunch of flowers instead. We did not observe any headteacher's request to governors for more pay being met by a similar gesture.

Our careful analysis of the interactions in formal governing body meetings indicated that, except where women held either or both of the roles of headteacher or chairperson of the governing body, women spoke less than men and made shorter interventions (Deem, 1994c; Deem *et al.*, 1995). We also noted the silences of some governors in formal meetings; these invariably included women as well as ethnic minority and working-class governors of both sexes. Where the silent governors were women, they were often those who had a good knowledge of the day-to-day running of the school, something lacked by many of the far more vocal white male middle-class governors (Deem, 1990).

We also found that governing bodies did not very often concern themselves with matters to do with equal opportunities, whether this was about the achievements of girls and boys, the extent to which money intended for pupils with special needs was actually spent on those students, the respective promotion prospects of women and men staff, or the operation and monitoring of school policies on sexism, racism and sexual or racial harassment. In our first questionnaire these were not issues identified by most respondents as areas where they required training. The increase in the numbers of lay people on governing bodies and the enhancement of their formal responsibilities have been heralded across the United Kingdom as evidence of an increase in parent power. Yet parents include single and lesbian mothers as well as those living as heterosexual couples, working-class people as well as those from the middle and upper classes, and those from ethnic minority as well as ethnic majority groups. There is so far little evidence from UK studies to suggest that all these different kinds of parents have been empowered by the reforms (Adler *et al.*, 1994; McKeown, 1994). There is every indication that middle-class, well-educated, hetero-sexual, married, White parents and their children have been the main beneficiaries of the changes made to schools.

Women in the educational workforce

Educational institutions are not establishments composed of compliant staff and students who simply have restructuring imposed on them. Following Giddens, it is important to see everyone as a knowledgeable actor, rather than viewing organisa-tional structure and human agency as separable entities (Giddens, 1984). Further-more, as Ham and Hill note, policy is not best studied by assuming that it is first constructed by the powerful and then simply implemented (Ham and Hill, 1984). This represents a misunderstanding of what constitutes policy. What happens to social policy after its initial formulation is as much a part of the policy process as the legislation which gives it statutory force. In the space available it is not possible to give a comprehensive account of the ways in which women teachers and educational support staff have been affected by educational reforms; others have also found this daunting (Darley, 1993). I have therefore selected three themes involving women teachers, women headteachers or aspirants to such posts, and women support staff in schools.

In order to consider the first theme, the spotlight is turned on women primary-school teachers, since women dominate primary teaching throughout the United Kingdom (Government Statistical Services, 1993). In England, Wales and North-ern Ireland, women primary teachers have been particularly affected by that el-ement of school and curricular reform which has insisted that they must teach science as well as maths, reading and writing. Thus women whose own science education was often inadequate are now expected, with relatively little training or support, to teach children to be confident and proficient in science. Secondly, the work of Pollard *et al.* suggests that many primary teachers in England, many of whom, as we have noted, are women, have subverted some of the reforms to the curriculum and assessment by adapting these to their existing practices (Pollard *et al.*, 1994). The notion that women are the passive recipients of social policy is certainly not supported by such research. Women teachers are also likely to be affected by the greater financial instability which many primary and secondary schools have experienced as a result of changes to the way they are funded, since so much depends on pupil recruitment which cannot be assumed to follow a consistent pattern year in year out. One consequence of this may be a greater proliferation of temporary and fixed-term contracts, which increase the flexibility of labour in schools but also have consequences for women's employment patterns, since the majority of part-time teachers in the United Kingdom are women. As Acker notes, flexibility does not operate in women's favour if they end up in insecure and poorly remunerated posts (Acker, 1992b).

As far as women headteachers are concerned, the reforms have had other consequences. With the advent of local management of schools, being able to deal with budgets and finances as well as managing teaching and learning has become a central requirement of headteacher posts, affecting both those already in post and those who apply for such posts. Richardson, in a small-scale study of the job and person specifications for the post of secondary headships, found that financial expertise was a major feature (Richardson, 1993). It might reasonably be argued that women are just as likely to have financial expertise as men; however, there are a number of other factors which need to be taken into account here. Firstly, since, as noted earlier, male governors are often more predominant on governing bodies than women, and since the reforms have included giving lay governors more power over appointments to schools, this is a significant factor in the hiring of headteachers. The predominantly White membership of governing bodies may well also militate against the employment of female or male ethnic minority headteachers. We noticed both of these factors at work in the headship selection processes observed during our governing body research.

Secondly, as Acker's work has shown, women headteachers, especially those in primary schools, are particularly likely to see teaching and learning rather than finance as major concerns of their jobs (Acker, 1992a, 1992b). Thirdly, even where women do have financial expertise, not only may those appointing them not necessarily take this into account but, given the more accidental nature of women headteachers' careers (Evetts, 1990), it is less likely that they have undergone formal training in finance or other management skills. This is despite the fact that many women have considerable experience of managing children and households, including budgets, all of which can add a valuable dimension to their formal qualifications and experience of working in schools (Green, 1993).

The third way in which women who work in schools may be affected is by the way in which the local management aspects of educational reforms relate to women support staff. Many UK schools rely heavily on the work done by full- or part-time school secretaries, who are almost always women. Since the advent of local management, the role of school secretaries and other staff in similar roles has undergone dramatic change. Much of the day-to-day administration of the financial affairs of schools as well as allocation of resources and personnel matters is undertaken by school secretaries, as Reynolds' work in London schools demonstrates (Reynolds, 1993). However, they are often poorly paid and receive little formal public recognition of their key role. They may do the book-keeping side of financial delegation but it is usually headteachers and chairpersons of governing bodies who appear as the public face of financial management in schools and who make major decisions about resource allocation (Broadbent and Laughlin, 1993; Broadbent *et al.*, 1993). The recent educational reforms have thus made considerable impact on the careers and lives of many of the women employed in educational establishments; that impact is not necessarily in line with the doctrine of diversity and choice.

Conclusion

In this chapter I have looked at some of the differences and similarities between educational reform across different countries within the United Kingdom, noting that although there are considerable variations between England, Wales, Scotland and Northern Ireland, there are nevertheless some effects with respect to gender which are likely to be similar in whichever country they occur. Although, as I noted at the beginning, recent feminist theories have urged us not to examine gender differences *per se* but to explore the different positions and identities taken by women, this omits the possibility that there are still systematic modes of discrimination experienced by social categories and distinct patternings which relate to gender as well as to other dimensions of social equality. Thus whilst it is important to be aware of diversity in the positive sense, particularly in relation to membership of ethnic minority groups, sexual orientation and identity, age, life style and so on, we should beware of losing sight of the concept of equality in a more general sense. Education reforms in the United Kingdom, supposedly motivated by concerns to do with choice and greater consumer involvement as well as diversity, seem to have taken none of these seriously as far as women are concerned.

Although some elements of the reforms, including adoption of national curricula, may have some positive effects for women, the examples I have used – diversity as defined in official government discourse about school restructuring, sex education, lay involvement in education reform and women staff in educational establishments – all suggest that this is far from being the case for the education reforms as a whole. Perhaps, however, the most optimistic sign is to be found in the work of researchers and practitioners like Acker and Harris, who suggest that women are capable of creating their own female-centred culture in educational organisations and subverting policies so that they become favourable to the achievements of girls and women, however hostile the conditions under which they work (Acker, 1992a; Harris, 1994). This is indeed one of the unintended consequences of the education reform process and arguably the most important lesson to be derived from this analysis of women and recent educational reform policy.

Note

1. Two Equal Opportunities Commission funded research projects, one under the direction of Miriam David, Madeleine Arnot and Gaby Weiner at South Bank University, London, and the other carried out by Sally Brown and Sheila Riddell at the University of Stirling, are currently examining some of the effects of the British educational reforms on equal opportunities. They are due to report during 1995.

7 · Women and health care

Peggy Foster

Health care is predominantly a woman's world. On the one hand, women are the main providers of health care in our society; not only do women provide vast amounts of unpaid and often unrecognised health care within the family, they also form the majority of paid health care providers. On the other hand, women are the main consumers of health care services. In the mid-1980s women comprised 51 per cent of the UK population but consumed between 60 and 65 per cent of all NHS resources (OHE, 1987). Women visit their GP almost twice as often as men; consume more drugs and medicines than men, occupy hospital beds more than men and are admitted to psychiatric units more often then men (see Kane, 1991). Given such figures, it is perhaps surprising that men have not complained that the NHS allocates its resources unfairly in relation to gender. Probably most men assume, as do most health care analysts, that women have an innate need for their larger share of health care resources.

A growing body of critics of modern medicine, however, including a number of feminists, strongly question the assumption that women need ever increasing amounts of health care. These critics claim that much health care currently consumed by women actually does them more harm that good. In this chapter four key feminist criticisms of the current British health care system are presented: first, that women as health care providers are discriminated against within the health care system; second, that an ever expanding health care system is exerting more and more control over women's lives without solving their real health problems; third, that health care providers frequently display patriarchal, sexist and sometimes racist attitudes towards women patients which seriously affect many women's access to and use of health care services; fourth, that much conventional medical care is far less effective and more harmful than most women have been led to believe.

Women as health care providers

Women represent just under 80 per cent of the total NHS workforce, yet few women hold positions of power and authority within the health care system. In 1991 only 15 per cent of all consultant posts and only 3 per cent of consultant posts in surgical specialties were held by women, and women held only 18 per cent of general manager posts (Goss and Brown, 1991). Only three of the first 57 NHS trusts were chaired by a woman (National Association of Health Authorities and Trusts). In 1987 the National Steering Group on Equal Opportunities for Women concluded that:

> It could be assumed that the NHS would offer conditions of employment commensurate with its dependence on female talent for delivery of care to patients. Such an assumption would unfortunately be incorrect. . . . The NHS expects the majority of its workforce to conform to the working life patterns of the minority. Women are expected to work full-time without any breaks in their working lives, and if they cannot do this (for instance when caring for children) they are penalised by losing prospects of promotion, income and sometimes their jobs (as happens when they cannot return to work at specified hours). (National Steering Group on Equal Opportunities for Women, 1987)

Seven years later a report of an equality audit, commissioned by the North West Regional Health Authority, strongly suggested that, at least as far as women hospital doctors were concerned, virtually nothing had changed. This report concluded that NHS hospitals in the early 1990s were dominated by a male medical tradition which did not accept or welcome women doctors as full and equal colleagues. The report's authors described a 'discouragement culture' which not only discriminated against women – and ethnic minorities – but also created a strong resistance to change. This resistance was far more influential than any official equal-opportunity policies which were being adopted by the Department for Health. One consultant interviewed by the audit team openly admitted that the inflexible working practices which dominate hospital specialties protected men's careers:

> I think the inflexible practices are useful to some in that they cut out 50 per cent of the competition – i.e. women, early in their careers. This is why change is difficult. Some think the old ways are best precisely because they protect jobs. (Maddock and Parkin, 1994: 11)

The women doctors interviewed for this audit believed that it would be extremely difficult to reach consultant level and have children. One Senior House Officer commented 'I can't see myself having a family and being a Registrar.' The audit report questioned whether women would continue to choose a career in hospital medicine if it continued to be so incompatible with family life and children, and concluded: 'Women doctors will continue to leave hospital specialties such as obstetrics and gynaecology if working conditions and hours do not improve and flexible training is not introduced for all training grades' (Maddock and Parkin, 1994: 70).

General practice is usually assumed to be a softer career option for doctors than hospital medicine, but recent changes to general practitioners' contracts have actually made it more difficult for women to become full partners within a practice. In 1991 a *British Medical Journal* editorial commented on the mismatch between the government's stated wish to see an increase in the number of women GPs and its creation of new conditions of work which made it harder for women to work as full-time GPs. The editorial also cited recent studies which found that women still felt discriminated against when applying for posts in general practice (Hayden, 1991).

Although the number of women entering medical school is now, for the first time ever, slightly higher than the number of men, medicine has traditionally been a male profession. Ironically, however, studies have demonstrated that women even find it relatively difficult to get promoted in the traditionally all-female profession of nursing. A 1986 study found that male nurses were to be found disproportionately in nursing manager grades (Davies and Rosser, 1986). In one health district men comprised just 8 per cent of the total nursing labour force but 37 per cent of posts of nursing officer or above. The average time taken for nurses to progress from an initial qualification to a nursing officer grade was 8.4 years for men but 17.9 years for women. Yet these men did not have better qualifications than the women. The researchers found that managers denied that they discriminated against women when selecting candidates for managerial posts but that women with domestic commitments were seen as problematic and that men were both confident in putting themselves forward for promotion and 'informally encouraged to do so'. The researchers concluded that the climate within the NHS was 'hostile to women' and that it was this overall climate rather than any lack of ambition on the part of female nurses which seriously hampered their careers (Davies and Rosser, 1986).

Although women are still far from equal with men in relation to reaching the top within the NHS, there is at least a great deal of official concern and activity around this problem. Far less official concern has been shown, however, about racial inequalities within the NHS. Significantly, whilst we at least have national statistics on the proportion of women in various posts within the NHS, national statistics on the numbers and proportions of ethnic minority women in NHS posts were simply not available in the early 1990s. A few research studies, however, have indicated that Black women may find it doubly hard to succeed in climbing to the top of NHS hierarchies. The equality audit of women hospital doctors in the North Western Region interviewed a number of Black women doctors who reported being discriminated against because of their race. Eighty-six per cent of the women questioned thought that Black doctors were much more likely to face discrimination than women within the NHS (Maddock and Parkin, 1994). One Asian woman stated 'Although I hold a postgraduate degree and membership in O & G, because of my colour I am never considered for a credible post. For routine donkey-work, yes.' A medical staffing officer commented that the criteria used to select applicants for top posts were 'to be white, male, Manchester graduates' (Maddock and Parkin, 1994: 55). Studies have also found discrimination against Black women within nursing. In 1990 a King's Fund Equal Opportunities Task Force reported that racial inequality was widespread and deep-seated within nursing. It found that Black nurses were concentrated in enrolled nurse grades and on night shifts, and that ethnic minority nurses did not have equal access to training and career development opportunities (King's Fund, 1990). The Chair of the Royal College of Nursing's (RCN) race and ethnicity sub-committee recently stated

> Black or ethnic minority nurses are often greatly over qualified for positions and even then do not get opportunities for promotion. It is very common to find black and minority ethnic nurses who have studied and worked alongside their white colleagues see these white nurses become their managers. (George, 1994: 20)

Equal opportunities policies within the NHS have been framed within a strong tradition which emphasises fair competition between different groups for very limited high-status and high-paid posts. No official concern is being expressed about the very large numbers of women who never even reach the first rung of health care career ladders. These women, who are overwhelmingly working class and/or Black, work as cleaners, caterers and laundresses for NHS establishments and have always been low-paid. However, since compulsory competitive tendering for NHS ancillary services was introduced in 1983 many of these women have suffered pay cuts, worsening terms and conditions of work and redundancies even when contracts have been awarded to 'in-house' bidders (Milne, 1989). These women will certainly not benefit from high-profile projects such as Opportunity 2000. Feminist health policy analysts should, at the very least, point out that the working conditions and pay of these women health care providers is just as much a feminist social policy issue as the career opportunities afforded to far more privileged women doctors, managers and high-flying nurses.

The increasing medicalisation of women's lives

Most health care providers assume that the key to improving women's health lies in an ever expanding health care system. A great deal of time and energy is now spent by health care providers in persuading women to avail themselves of health care services. Whereas twenty or so years ago, the health care system tended simply to wait for women to come forward and ask for advice or treatment, the current system is far more proactive. Many GPs, for example, now actively pursue their female patients to ensure that they receive regular cervical smear tests (see Ross, 1989). Women who refuse to respond to such pressure may even risk being crossed off their GP's list. In

November 1990 *The Guardian* reported that one GP had threatened to strike twenty women off his list on the grounds that their refusal to have a smear test was costing his practice £1,300 of government reward monies for meeting screening targets (*The Guardian*, 28 November 1990).

Whereas cervical screening has expanded over many years in an unplanned and haphazard fashion, the national breast cancer screening programme was very carefully planned and co-ordinated from its inception. As part of that planning, a great deal of health promotion literature was produced in order to encourage older women to take up the offer of a breast screening test or mammography. Despite a remarkably good response to these offers, British women have already been blamed by a number of medical experts for putting the success of early breast cancer screening programmes at risk by failing to attend for screening in adequate numbers (see, for example, Roberts *et al.*, 1990).

The cervical and breast cancer screening programmes have created a lot of extra work for health care providers and have also no doubt boosted the profits of the manufacturers of screening equipment and the equipment used in the treatment of those women whose screening tests prove positive. Despite some complaints of over-work by laboratory staff, medical screening has thus clearly been of benefit to those who make their living from providing health care. What these programmes clearly fail to do, however, is to tackle the primary causes of breast and cervical cancer. For example, the strong possibility of a link between industrial pollutants and a high risk of cervical cancer (see Robinson, 1981) has received virtually no attention from health care providers who continue to insist – despite very disappointing results (see McPherson and Savage, 1987) – that a well-organised screening programme is the most effective approach to preventing cervical cancer.

The continuing expansion of the medicalisation of women's lives is by no means limited to health prevention activities. New medical treatments for what were pre-viously regarded as natural life events or unalterable misfortunes are also being heavily promoted within the current health care system. For example, during the 1950s and 1960s, British doctors' attitudes to the menopause were that it was a natural life event which caused 'normal' women very few real problems. Jeffcoate's *Principles of Gynaecology* claimed in 1957, for example, 'In the well adjusted and well informed woman psychological changes [during the menopause] are few and insignifi-cant' (Jeffcoate, 1957: 93). By the 1990s, however, a new medical consensus on the menopause was emerging which viewed it primarily as a hormone deficiency disease from which all older women suffered (see, for example, Gangar and Key, 1991). More and more British doctors are now treating menopausal women with some form of hormone replacement therapy (HRT) (Audit Commission, 1994). One British gynaecologist has even claimed that post-menopausal women would be much better off having a total hysterectomy followed by HRT than hanging on to their redundant wombs. According to Studd:

Usually when women have a hysterectomy and then take oestrogen therapy alone, they say they haven't felt so well for years and wonder why they didn't have it before. There's every advantage in having the womb plus ovaries removed and then having hormone therapy forever. (Studd, 1988: 68)

Whilst many older women have very strongly endorsed HRT as the solution to all their menopausal problems (see e.g. Cooper, 1979), others, including a number of prominent feminists, have pointed out that HRT will have no impact on the social and economic causes of older women's distress (see Ussher, 1989). The commercial and medical promotion of HRT encourages older women to seek a medical elixir of youth rather than to challenge the sexist and ageist attitudes which lead our society to devalue and discount middle-aged women whilst admiring more powerful middle-aged men.

Another quite dramatic example of the increasing medicalisation of women's lives is the growth of 'high-tech' infertility treatments. Thirty years ago modern medicine had very little to offer women who failed to conceive naturally. Today such women can hope to be helped by very sophisticated medical techniques such as *in vitro* fertilisation (IVF) and gamete intra fallopian transfer (GIFT). These expensive and still relatively unsuccessful treatments are not easily obtainable within the NHS (*The Lancet*, 1993) but are readily available to those couples who can afford to pay for them. Whilst these high-technology medical solutions to infertility have attracted a great deal of attention both within the health care system and from the media, the primary causes of infertility remain under-researched and under-treated.

Throughout their adult lives women are now encouraged to use a whole range of health care services, even when they are perfectly well. Young women are encouraged to use medicalised forms of contraception such as the pill. Later on, during their reproductive years, women are often either subject to close medical scrutiny during pregnancy or pulled into high-technology infertility treatment programmes. As they grow older women are likely to be offered psychotropic drugs for the depression and anxiety that often accompany marriage and motherhood and then HRT for any anxiety associated with the menopausal years. By the time they reach old age a very high proportion of women will be taking some type of prescribed drug or medicine and many women will again be medically treated for the stress-related symptoms which accompany the low-status and low-income years of later life (Burns and Phillipson, 1986). Meanwhile the underlying social and economic factors which play such an important role in determining women's health status and health-related problems receive very little attention from a society still apparently convinced that increasing expenditure on an ever expanding health care empire is the best way to improve the health of the nation.

Doctors' attitudes towards women

Feminist critics of patriarchal health care systems have repeatedly exposed the extent to which health care providers hold views and assumptions about women in general and certain 'types' of women in particular which are detrimental to women's experiences of health care. For example, Ann Oakley's study of pregnant women's experiences of ante-natal care and childbirth demonstrated that doctors frequently discount women's own knowledge about their own bodies, their lives and their health care needs (Oakley, 1980). Oakley gives a classic example of this tendency in the form of a brief interaction between a doctor and a pregnant woman during an ante-natal clinic.

DOCTOR (reading case notes): Ah, I see you've got a boy and a girl.
PATIENT: No, two girls.
DOCTOR: Really, are you sure? I thought it said . . . [checks in case notes] oh no, you're quite right, two girls.

(Oakley, 1980: 41)

Not all examples of doctors ignoring women's own experiences are as amusing as this one. Women reporting quite serious side effects whilst using prescribed drugs have recounted how their doctors simply took no notice of them. This appears to be a particularly common occurrence in relation to women's reporting of the side effects of the pill. Research carried out in the early 1980s into the experiences of middle-class women taking the pill found that doctors tended to take little notice of women's experiences of side effects. One woman, for example, reported: 'It was as if I was imagining them. . . . It's almost as though they can't hear you' (Pollock, 1984: 146).

One of the reasons why doctors may ignore women's complaints about the unpleasant side effects of medical treatments is that many doctors still appear to regard women as innately more neurotic and prone to emotional instability than men. The medical profession's view of women as innately mentally unstable has a long history. In the late nineteenth century an exclusively male medical profession pronounced women to be totally governed by their wombs and subject to the uniquely female maladies of hysteria and neurasthenia (Ussher, 1989). As Ussher has pointed out, doctors no longer believe in these complaints but they do believe in modern versions of female madness such as pre-menstrual syndrome, post-natal depression and menopausal anxiety. Thus women consulting their GPs with symptoms of anxiety or depression may well be told 'It's just your age' or 'It's a hormonal imbalance' when they themselves know all too well that they are primarily responding to family, work or money problems. Researchers who have interviewed women suffering from anxiety and depression have found that many of these women have not been happy with their doctors' explanations of their problem. One woman in Agnes Miles' study commented, for example: 'Dr D just said it was my age and the change. I told him I did't think it was because I still have periods. . . . He is an efficient doctor but he doesn't like nerve cases' (Miles, 1988: 120). Another woman cited by Corob explained:

I was told I had an endogenous depression which I found out later was a depression that comes out of the blue and has no obvious cause. Well I felt the cause was obvious. I had plenty of explanations for it. But they just thought I was over reacting I suppose. (Corob, 1987: 11)

Whilst many doctors still appear to hold rather patronising, if not patriarchal, views about women in general, they also tend to make assumptions about their female patients based on particular social factors such as the patient's age, class and ethnic background. Black women, for example, have reported how White male doctors have categorised them as unsuitable for motherhood and unreliable in relation to the control of their own fertility. One Afro-Caribbean woman who experienced very bad side effects from the pill asked her family-planning clinic if she could try a low-dose pill but she found that:

> I really had to put up a fight to get them to prescribe it for me. You know why? Because it was a low dosage pill and they didn't think I was responsible enough to take it regularly at the same time every day. (Bryan *et al.*, 1985: 102)

Bryan *et al.* have written:

> Because we are considered a 'high promiscuity risk' black and white working class women are often encouraged to accept contraceptives involving less 'risk' – but the reduced risk of pregnancy is invariably considered more important than the increased risk to our health. And so we are prescribed a coil, which can infect our fallopian tubes . . . or Depo-Provera which can have dangerous, long-term side effects. (Bryan *et al.*, 1985: 102)

Women living in poverty may also receive particularly controlling types of medical advice. For example, Reid advises doctors in *Handbook of Family Planning* that for poorly motivated women

> who include the mothers of large families, of children in care or with very little care, those with haphazard personal and social relationships, in trouble with the law, and with substandard living conditions . . . methods such as the IUD or the injectable which do not require the patients' cooperation are often best. (Reid, 1985: 36)

Health providers' highly judgemental attitudes towards certain types of female patients do not just affect the medical advice which they are given. Judgemental or prejudicial attitudes can also play a crucial role in determining women's access to a range of medical services. For example, doctors are highly selective when determining which women will be given access to NHS-based IVF and GIFT programmes. As well as selecting only those women whom they regard as physically suitable for such treatment, doctors also make judgements about women's social suitability for parenthood. For example, in order to get on to the waiting list of an NHS-based IVF clinic in Manchester a woman must have lived with a male partner for at least three years and the couple must fulfil adoption criteria (Douglas *et al.*, 1992). In 1987 a guide to infertility treatment published by the BMA asked 'Can a single woman ask for IVF?' and replied:

She can ask but most units will refuse her. Many feminist groups feel that it is a woman's right to have a child when she wants and in the way she wants, but society and clinicians find it difficult to offer such an expensive, complex, and extremely demanding treatment to single women while 12% or more of stable couples are trying so hard to have children to bring up within the family. (Leila and Elliot, 1987: 10)

Doctors selecting women for IVF or GIFT are quite overtly making judgements about their suitability for motherhood based on social norms (or prejudice) which have nothing whatever to do with clinical decision making. In this sense doctors can be said to be exerting social control over women on behalf of a patriarchal society which only regards women as suitable for motherhood if they are firmly attached to an affluent male partner. Ironically, women who are deemed suitable mothers by the medical profession may face difficulties gaining access to NHS abortions or sterilisation on the grounds that they ought to be fulfilling their duty as suitable mothers (see Aitken-Swan, 1977) and do not therefore altogether avoid the negative consequences of doctors' patriarchal attitudes.

Whilst all women may be subject to doctors' patriarchal attitudes, women from the ethnic minorities also frequently have to face overt racism within the health care system. One young Black woman has recounted her experience of giving birth in an NHS hospital thus:

I think when you are young and go to hospital to have a baby, they should be more helpful, more concerned. This sister said to me, 'You black people have too many babies.' As far as I was concerned, I wasn't 'You black people', I was me. You don't forget something like that. Even now it makes me angry to think about it. I don't see what business she has to say that, she was supposed to be caring for me. (Larbie, 1985: 19)

Asian women have also reported some very negative experiences of maternity care, partly due to overt racism by individual health care providers, but also due to institutional indifference to their particular needs, especially their need to be communicated with in a language they fully understand. For example, one Asian woman interviewed by Jean Hennings explained that her young daughter had had to translate the information given to her after an ultrasound scan indicated that her baby had died in the womb and that she would have to undergo an immediate termination. Only when her daughter could no longer understand what was being said was an interpreter called. Another Asian woman recounted that on her first ante-natal clinic visit during her seventh pregnancy, a male doctor had asked her angrily: 'How many children? How many do you want? 10, 15, 20, 25? You have got enough.' She explained: 'I couldn't say anything. I don't speak English. I couldn't tell him that God has sent me my children. . . . Hospitals don't like us, we have so many children' (Hennings, 1993: 15).

Most health authorities have now introduced some system for providing link workers or translators for pregnant Asian women who speak little English, but according to Randhawa, a typical attitude expressed by maternity care providers is: 'You don't need to be able to talk to a mother to deliver a baby' (Randhawa, 1986: 9).

In the late 1970s and early 1980s many local health authorities provided English lessons for pregnant Asian women (Maternity Alliance, 1985). This idea may sound reasonable until we consider how an English woman might fare if she found herself pregnant in Japan and was offered six hours or so of Japanese lessons to enable her to understand a Japanese-speaking obstetric team.

Doctors working in overstretched NHS hospitals may have little time to communicate effectively with any of their patients, but according to obstetrician Wendy Savage, the problem of doctor–patient communication is not just one of lack of time. She found that when registrars became members of her ante-natal team and were given a reasonable amount of time for each appointment, they actually did not know how to use it all since they were so 'unused to letting the woman express her fears and concerns and spending time on discussing these' (Savage, 1991: 884). Affluent middle-class women who object to doctors treating them in a dismissive or patronising way do now have some choice over their response. A few brave souls may challenge their doctors and insist that they answer their questions fully and openly, but even the most articulate and confident women have reported feeling disempowered when lying on a medical couch being examined by a consultant gynaecologist who discusses their problem with them whilst they still have their legs in the air.

Another option for affluent women is to turn for help with their health problems to the private or alternative health care sector. Health care commentators frequently express their concern about inequalities within the NHS such as the fact that younger middle-class women are more likely to have regular smear tests than older working-class women (e.g. Townsend and Davidson, 1992: 74). However, to date little attention appears to have been paid to the extent to which affluent women buy access to complementary medicine as an alternative to the mainstream health care system. There has been an extraordinary growth in alternative or complementary health care services such as aromatherapy, acupuncture, homeopathy, reflexology, remedial massage, herbalism – to name but a few – but as this whole system is still remarkably unregulated we do not know – although we can guess – the extent to which its clientele is predominantly White, middle class and female. We do know that affluent women buy more conventional private health care services, particularly private abortions, and that one of their reasons for doing so is that they feel they will be treated more sympathetically within the private sector (Clarke *et al.*, cited by Higgins, 1988).

Middle-class women are also buying themselves the privilege of a home birth using private midwifery services. According to Ann Oakley, the home birth movement in Britain has promoted a situation in which

> people with money can buy themselves out of the rundown, disadvantaged and undoubtedly at times inflexible NHS and into a private alternative which suits them better. Here, women can obtain the kind of birth they want simply by dint of paying for it. (Oakley, 1987: 27)

Those mainstream health providers and medical experts who are highly critical of many of the alternative health care interventions have claimed that one major problem with such services is their lack of scientific credibility. They have accused alternative practitioners of failing to prove scientifically that their therapies are effective (see Skrabanek and McCormick, 1989). Yet there is growing evidence that much mainstream medicine is less effective than many doctors and their female patients believe. There is also a large body of evidence on the negative side effects of many mainstream medical interventions. There is not the space to explore all of this evidence in this chapter but in the following section we will examine just two key areas of modern medicine which are less effective than many women assume: ante-natal care and breast cancer screening and treatment.

The ineffectiveness of modern medicine

Routine ante-natal tests

Many pregnant women have told researchers that attending hospital-based ante-natal clinics is rarely a congenial experience. Women have complained that such clinics are frequently overcrowded, tedious and impersonal. They have also reported that asking for advice and reassurance in a hospital-based clinic is extremely difficult (National Childbirth Trust, 1991).

Yet, despite these complaints, very few women fail to attend for routine ante-natal check-ups. Presumably most women strongly believe that not attending would put their own health and the health of their unborn child at risk. Certainly this is the message that women receive from 'the experts'. The very widely read booklet produced by the Health Education Authority (HEA) entitled *Pregnancy Book* advises women, for example: 'the earlier you go [for ante-natal care] the better. If there is anything wrong, however slight, then it's best to find out early so the problem can be dealt with' (HEA, 1991: 27).

What most pregnant women are not told, and therefore cannot know, is that there is now a growing body of dissent within the medical and nursing professions which challenges the dominant view that ante-natal care plays a major role in reducing perinatal and maternal mortality and morbidity. Indeed some medical experts have now gone so far as to suggest that many of the routine checks performed on all pregnant women during ante-natal visits are a waste of time and resources. In September 1993 an editorial in the *British Medical Journal*, for example, argued that the rituals of weighing women in early pregnancy, testing their urine for glucose and listening for a foetal heartbeat were all of little or no value as screening devices (Steer, 1993). Not only are these procedures now questioned as accurate diagnostic tools, but there is also evidence that, despite being simple and non-invasive, such tests may unnecessarily cause some women acute stress. If a woman is identified during routine ante-natal care as failing to put on enough weight, for example, the consequences for her may be quite unpleasant. One woman has reported: 'I dreaded going to the clinic because I knew they would go on about my weight.' When this woman reached her estimated delivery date she was offered an elective Caesarian but gave birth to a very normal 6lb 4oz daughter. She commented: 'I really didn't mind about the Caesarian. By that time I was so terrified that my baby wasn't getting enough food and so miserable that I just wanted the pregnancy to be over' (Howarth, 1991: 57).

Whilst some of the routine simple tests carried out on millions of pregnant women may be less safe and efficacious than was once thought, most critical attention in recent years has focused on the new more 'high-tech' screening procedure of ultra-sound. Ultrasound was first developed during the Second World War to track down enemy submarines. Medical ultrasound scanning began to be used as a diagnostic aid in high-risk pregnancies during the 1970s but by the late 1980s it was routinely used in most ante-natal clinics. Most obstetricians are convinced that ultrasound is a safe procedure which, in expert hands, can provide a whole range of useful information from determining the exact age of the foetus to checking for multiple births and foetal position and to indicating some types of foetal abnormalities. A number of critics of ultrasound, on the other hand, have expressed a range of concerns over its ever increasing use in routine ante-natal care. According to its critics, ultrasound scanning is a major form of medical experimentation which has never been subjected to the type of clinical trials which would be necessary to rule out any long-term harmful effects of its wide-scale use. The Association for Improvements in Maternity Service (AIMS), for example, 'strongly question the ethics of exposing the majority of children born in this country to a potentially dangerous procedure whose long term effects have not been adequately researched' (AIMS, 1991: 486).

In 1993 a report in *The Lancet* of the Perth randomised controlled trial of frequent pre-natal ultrasound examinations concluded that frequent ultrasound scans appeared to be associated with low birthweight and concluded: 'it is . . . plausible that frequent exposure to ultrasound may have influenced fetal growth' (Newnham *et al.*, 1993: 887).

Whilst any possible long-term risks associated with routine ultrasound testing remain at present very largely hypothetical, the more immediate risks of ultrasound are well proven. For example, the risk of ultrasound falsely detecting some type of foetal abnormality is a real one. One study from Harvard showed that among 3,100 scans, eighteen babies were erroneously picked out as abnormal (McTaggart, 1990). In the most extreme cases such misdiagnoses by ultrasound can lead to a pregnant woman opting to abort an apparently abnormal foetus which proves to have been perfectly normal. AIMS gave evidence to the House of Commons Health Committee, stating that they knew of a number of cases where this had happened (AIMS, 1991: 486).

If routine ultrasound scanning clearly carries some risk of wrong diagnosis and concomitant anxiety and distress to the pregnant woman thus tested, are such costs nevertheless outweighed by the benefits it brings? Not according to the American College of Obstetrics and Gynaecology in 1984, which stated: 'No well-controlled study [had yet] proved that routine screening of prenatal patients will improve the outcome of pregnancy' (McTaggart, 1990: 2).

In 1993 the authors of a meta-analysis of randomised trials evaluating the effect of routine ultrasound scanning involving 15,935 pregnancies concluded:

> Routine ultrasound scanning does not improve the outcome of pregnancy in terms of an increased number of the live births or of reduced perinatal mortality. Routine ultrasound scanning may be effective and useful as a screening for malformation. Its use for this purpose, however, should be made explicit and take into account the risk of false positive diagnosis in addition to ethical issues. (Bucher and Schmidt, 1993: 13)

On balance, therefore, it appears that the case for routine ante-natal tests, including ultrasound screening is not as strong as many health care providers and pregnant women believe, and that there is at least some evidence to suggest that these routine tests occasionally inflict serious harm on both pregnant women and their unborn children.

Breast cancer screening and treatment

In 1987, just before a general election, the government announced that it was going to fund one of the first national breast-screening programmes which would invite all women aged between 50 and 64 for mammographic screening at three-yearly intervals. According to the government's *The Health of the Nation*, the aim of this programme is now 'to reduce breast cancer deaths in the population invited for screening by 25% by 2000 compared to 1990' (Secretary of State for Health, 1991). Given that the United Kingdom has the highest breast cancer mortality rate in the world – 52 deaths per 100,000 women – and that a British woman has a one in twelve chance of developing the disease (Faulder, 1993), this aim appears to be highly laudable. However, even many doctors are highly sceptical about the government's very optimistic target for reducing deaths from breast cancer (see, for example, Williams, 1991).

A number of critics of breast cancer screening have argued that on balance the national screening programme is likely to cause women more harm that good. This claim is partly based on several inherent weaknesses of breast screening by mammography. For example, mammograms are known to produce a relatively high number of false positive test results, which means that significant numbers of women screened will undergo the trauma of being called back for further tests (see Skrabanek, 1988; Rodgers, 1991) before being told that they do not after all have an early malignant tumour. Some critics of breast screening have also suggested that at least some of those tumours found through mammography will be so latent or slow growing that even without detection by mammogram they would pose no threat to a woman's life or well being (see Klemi *et al.*, 1992). There is even some concern that, far from reducing significantly deaths from breast cancer, widespread use of mammograms could actually increase the prevalence of this disease. According to Dr Michael

Swift, for example, some women's genetic make-up may make them particularly susceptible to developing breast cancer after being exposed to even extremely low doses of radiation (Swift *et al.*, 1991).

Despite all these known weaknesses of breast screening by mammography, the benefits of a national breast-screening programme might still quite clearly outweigh the costs if modern medicine could guarantee to cure all or even most early tumours detected by mammography. Unfortunately, such a cure remains to be discovered. All that breast cancer specialists can now offer is a variety of treatments which have been proved to reduce the risk of local recurrence of the disease and/or increase average length of survival from diagnosis.

Neither of these useful outcomes of treatment, however, can be regarded as a complete cure. Moreover, the standard form of treatment for breast cancer throughout the twentieth century – the mastectomy – has now been proved over and over again to be no more effective in prolonging women's lives than breast-conserving surgery such as lumpectomy. As early as just after the Second World War a clinical study demonstrated that radical mastectomies which involve removal of the chest wall as well as the breast itself did not significantly improve long-term survival rates when compared with less radical surgery. Similar research findings were published in the 1960s. Yet many surgeons continued to perform radical mastectomies to remove even relatively small tumours until well into the 1980s. In 1986 the *British Medical Journal* published the report from a Consensus Development Conference on the treatment of primary breast cancer (Consensus Development Conference, 1986). In this report a group of top breast cancer specialists concluded that there was no evidence that any type of mastectomy led to longer survival rates compared to local removal of the tumour or lumpectomy. Despite this accumulation of clear scientific evidence, some surgeons continue to offer women a mastectomy as the safest form of treatment for very small breast tumours. It is hard not to conclude from the long history of ineffective mastectomy surgery that this disabling and disfiguring treatment could only have been perpetuated within a health care system which pays far too much regard to the status, independence and individual clinical judgement of male surgeons and far too little regard to the physical and psychological pain and disability suffered by thousands upon thousands of breast cancer patients who have apparently lost their breasts unnecessarily.

If many women have been misled into believing that mastectomies are 'safer' than less radical forms of breast cancer surgery, they have also been misled into believing that the so-called adjuvant therapies for breast cancer such as chemotherapy and radiotherapy can cure them of this disease. For example, in 1991 readers of the *Daily Mirror* were informed by a consultant radiotherapist that the NHS did not have sufficient radiotherapy machines to treat and *cure* the increasing number of women being diagnosed as suffering from early breast cancer (*Daily Mirror*, 25 September 1991). Yet in 1986 the Consensus Development Conference stated baldly 'there is no evidence that radiotherapy prolongs life' (p. 946). It can prevent local recurrence of the disease, but specialists fully understand that this benefit is not the same as a 'cure'. Similarly the 1986 Conference concluded that chemotherapy could increase survival rates at five years for women under fifty but that 'any benefits are substantially less in women over 50' (p. 947). Finally the Conference reported that 'endocrine therapy with tamoxifen given for two years after initial treatment in patients over 50 results in both a reduced relapse rate and a reduction in death from 30% to 24% over five years'. For women under fifty, however, the Conference did not find convincing evidence of a reduction in mortality after treatment with tamoxifen (p. 947).

Having had at least some success with tamoxifen as a treatment for breast cancer, some specialists have been very keen to research the use of tamoxifen as a preventative agent in healthy women with a particularly high familial risk of developing breast cancer. Critics of this approach, however, have pointed out that the known risks of long-term tamoxifen use such as a significant increase in the risk of endometrial cancer, together with the unpleasant side effects experienced by many women who take tamoxifen, make it unsuitable as a drug to be taken by healthy cancer-free women (Fugh-Berman and Epstein, 1992). According to one such critic, there is a real risk that as 'doctors scramble on to the tamoxifen bandwagon' the harm done to healthy women by this drug will soon outweigh any possible reduction in breast cancer which it might produce (McTaggart, 1993).

Women with a genetically high risk of developing breast cancer have not only been identified as ideal subjects to test out the preventative potential of tamoxifen, they are also being seen as potential consumers of a new screening test for a 'breast cancer gene' which is currently being developed. Commercial companies are already preparing to market this test once the breast cancer gene has been identified. One researcher believes that 'there will be a commercial interest attached to seeing as many people screened as possible' (Brown, 1993). However, women who will be targeted to take this new test ought to be warned in advance that if the test were to prove positive the medical options available to them would not be attractive ones – to say the least. In the United States women in severely affected families have already opted to have 'prophylactic surgery' to prevent breast cancer – a clinical term for the removal of both breasts and sometimes both ovaries as well (Brown, 1993).

In 1994 an article in the *British Medical Journal* on familial breast cancer stated: 'An energetic attempt to reduce the risk of breast cancer would include the option of prophylactic bilateral mastectomy' (Evans *et al.*, 1994: 186). At a time in history when breast cancer specialists are finally accepting the evidence, which has been available to them for decades, that mastectomies do not prolong the lives of breast cancer patients compared to less radical forms of treatment, it is worrying to say the very least, that some doctors are now prepared to perform prophylactic mastectomies on perfectly healthy women.

Conclusion

The evidence presented in this chapter has indicated that the current health care system is failing women in at least four key ways. First, women health care providers are still far less likely to reach the top of the NHS hierarchy than their male counter-parts whether they are working as doctors, nurses or managers. Although the NHS has recently adopted a high-profile equal-opportunities policy in relation to its female employees there is as yet very little evidence that this policy is being fully imple-mented at ground level, or that the traditional medical culture which has for so long discriminated against women health care providers is in terminal decline.

Second, women as health care consumers are being subjected to ever increasing pressure to use an ever growing range of health care products and services even when they feel perfectly fit and well. Yet this increased medicalisation of women's lives fails to tackle the root causes of women's morbidity and mortality such as the poverty endured by a very significant number of women in our society.

Third, partly because the NHS is still very much a White male-dominated institu-tion, health care providers still display attitudes towards women in general, and certain groups of women in particular, which adversely affect women's access to, and use of, a whole range of health care services.

Fourth, modern medicine promises women far more than it can deliver. Women learn from an early age that there is a medical solution to virtually all their problems. Yet there is an impressive body of medical literature – not readily accessible to the lay reader – which strongly suggests that a whole range of medical interventions are less effective than women are generally led to believe. This means that women's overall health and well-being are far less dependent on their use of medical services than most health care providers claim. Moreover, many forms of medical intervention impose both physical and emotional damage on many of the women who consume them. Overall, therefore, an evaluation of the impact of the current health care system on women's lives must conclude that it meets far less of women's genuine health needs than is widely assumed.

8   *Women and the personal social services*

Ann Davis

Introduction

Personal social services are delivered to citizens deemed to be in need of them, by a mix of state, voluntary, private and informal agencies. The boundaries and the terrain of the territory of personal social services have changed over time in response to major legislative, social policy, organisational, political and economic imperatives. The personal social services are currently undergoing further transformation as a result of legislative change (particularly the Children Act 1989 and the National Health Service and Community Care Act 1990) as well as changes and proposed changes to the organisation of local government in England, Wales, Scotland and Northern Ireland. The personal social services have traditionally been an area of social policy and provision in which women have had a substantial presence as service users and front-line service providers.

This chapter focuses on why women's presence has been such a consistent feature of the personal social services and what the current changes to these services are likely to mean for women as service users and workers. In doing so, it is concerned to identify the gendered characteristics of this sphere of social policy and provision in Britain. To this end the first half of this chapter provides an account of the scope and organisation of the personal social services and the position of women as workers and service users. The second half of the chapter considers some of the assumptions about women which are embedded in the personal social services. It does this by exploring the official visions of the personal social services which have been promoted by government and the critiques of these visions which have been developed by feminist social policy and social work analysts.

The scope of the personal social services

Any consideration of this area of social policy and provision has to start with some account of what is meant by the term 'personal social services', as it has proved to be a difficult term to define. Several contributors to the literature on this subject (e.g. Sainsbury, 1975; Hallett, 1982, 1989; Webb and Wistow, 1987; Hill, 1993; Baldock, 1994) have offered interesting contributions to the debate regarding the delineation of the territory of the personal social services in Britain.

The term 'personal social services' is one which has a relatively recent history. Its adoption reflects the work undertaken in the late 1960s and early 1970s when the role and remit of local authority health and welfare activities were being reviewed by government. The outcome of this work was the creation of Social Service Departments in England and Wales and subsequently Social Work Departments in Scotland and Health and Welfare Boards in Ireland.

At its narrowest, the personal social services have been conceived as those services provided directly and indirectly (through voluntary and private organisations) by local authority Social Services Departments (SSDs) in England and Wales (see e.g. Hill, 1993). For others the term indicates a much wider remit.

> Responsibility for them spans a broad spectrum. At the centre are local authority social services departments. . . . Closely linked are district health authorities and family health service authorities, currently responsible for primary health care and community health care outside of the acute hospital sector. Social security, education, housing, police and courts and the probation service may be involved. There is also a rich diversity of service providers in the voluntary and private sectors. (DoH, 1994a: 9)

At its widest, the term has been used to refer to the sets of statutory, private, voluntary arrangements which are

> concerned with needs and difficulties which inhibit the individual's maximum social functioning, his [sic] freedom to develop his personality and to achieve his aspirations through relationships with others; needs which have been traditionally dealt with by personal and family action . . . needs for which we usually ascribe some individual responsibility in the helping process, rather than a uniformity of provision. . . . The personal social services are concerned with the individualisation of services, and with adjusting the use of certain

resources by individuals, families and groups, according to an assessment of their differential needs. (Sainsbury, 1975: 3)

Baldock has questioned the emphasis placed on the concept of 'need' in such definitions of the personal social services. He argues that:

> needs play a surprisingly small part in determining the scale and scope of the personal social services. Need, in the sense of numbers of people and their circumstances, is just one of the factors that decide personal social services provision. There are many other, often more important ingredients in the mix: changes in professional opinion and behaviour, decisions about local government organisation and finance, developments in other parts of the welfare system such as in housing and health services, press outcry when the negligent, cruel or unacceptable is discovered. (Baldock, 1994: 162)

Yet the 'language of need' is constantly used by politicians, professionals and the public in defining the personal social services.

Webb and Wistow also take issue with broad definitions such as Sainsbury's which, they argue, do little to capture the reality of the history and current range of responses made by the personal social services in Britain. The origins of the personal social services lie in the Poor Law response of the state as well as that of nineteenth-century philanthropic and voluntary organisations to the destitution of individuals and households who lacked the resources to maintain themselves and those who were dependent on them. In the post-war welfare state legislation the Poor Law was abolished and its functions were taken on by several health and local authority departments with a remit to provide services themselves or through voluntary and private organisations for children and families as well as older people and those with illness or disability (Webb and Wistow, 1987).

The Seebohm Report, which presented a review of the organisation and responsibilities of the local authority personal social services in England and Wales and the subsequent legislation (the Local Authority Social Services Act 1970), attempted to unify these services as a 'fifth' social service alongside the established social services of housing, income maintenance, health and education (Townsend, 1970). Like its counterparts, the personal social services reflected, and continue to reflect, a mixed economy of provision drawing on informal, private, voluntary and statutory sources. In contrast to its counterparts the personal social services drew on relatively little public expenditure resourcing and continued to be a relatively 'poor relation' in public expenditure terms (see Figure. 8.1).

Webb and Wistow argue that in examining what constitutes the personal social services

> it is essential to accept and live with a broad, loose and ambiguous delineation of our field as consisting of all the work undertaken by SSDs with the addition

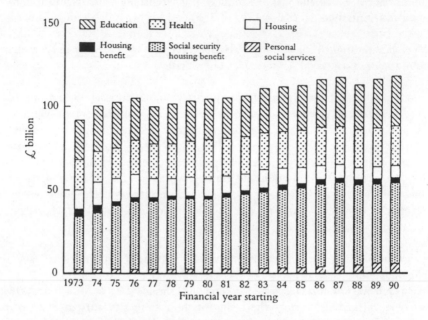

Figure 8.1 Public spending on welfare in the United Kingdom 1973–90 (1990–91 prices). (Source: Glennerster, 1992)

of all the activities within the informal, voluntary and private sectors which correspond broadly to the remit of the SSDs. (Webb and Wistow, 1987: 8)

The approach which this chapter adopts is to consider the territory of the personal social services in the terms outlined by Webb and Wistow. Those activities and tasks which fall within the scope of the personal social services are considered to be the distribution of a range of goods and services which individuals are routinely expected to provide for themselves and with assistance from family and friends. This range includes the care and control of children and adults, support of both an emotional and material kind when illness or disability strikes and basic domestic servicing.

These goods and services span personal care, domestic and maintenance services delivered to individuals' households, day care, residential accommodation offering respite from or a permanent substitute for home, investigation of the care provided for children and adults by members of their households, the removal of vulnerable children and adults from their households to substitute homes or other forms of accommodation, the provision of adaptations and equipment to households designed to increase the access and choices of disabled people, cash payments made directly or indirectly to individuals to secure a service or maintain the care of dependants.

This range of goods and services is made available to poor and excluded citizens facing crisis or deemed to be 'at risk' who are assessed as being deserving of assistance from the personal social services. Some of these citizens have actively sought intervention in their lives from the personal social services, some have had intervention thrust upon them. Amongst their ranks women predominate. This is the result of a number of interrelated factors. Women outnumber men amongst poor citizens in Britain (Glendinning and Millar, 1992). Women also outnumber men amongst the minority of those older citizens who receive help from the social services (Henwood, 1992). Critically too, women in Britain are designated as carrying prime responsibility for the care (and control) of children and other adults requiring help with personal care. As mothers, daughters, sisters and neighbours, women are far more likely than men to come to the attention of the personal social services for advice, assistance and assessment in relation to the way in which they carry out these responsibilities.

The administration and financing of the personal social services

There are considerable variations in the location of the administration of the personal social services in Britain. In 1994, in England and Wales 116 Social Services Departments had responsibility for personal social services. These were located in 33 London Boroughs, 36 Metropolitan Districts and 47 County Councils. In Scotland nine Social Work Departments (plus three island councils) provided a range of services which included work with offenders (probation and after-care). These departments were located at the regional tier of local government. In Northern Ireland the services were the responsibility of four appointed welfare and health boards. As a consequence of local government reviews the administration and organisation of the local authority personal social services in Britain is shaping up for further change.

Whatever the consequences of current changes in the administrative location of the personal social services the power which central government exercises in determining the resources available for the personal social services is unlikely to shift. As Baldock points out:

> Central government makes the essential decisions determining how much money will be available for the personal social services. But it makes them with only a broad and technical reference to social need. It also decides the duties and objectives of the services. Local authorities must do the best they can to fulfil their legal obligations within the funds made available to them. (Baldock, 1994: 162)

The resources which have been made available to local authorities over the last two decades for the personal social services reflect two periods of real growth. These periods are associated with the two major periods of legislative change, 1971–6 and 1986–92 (see Table 8.1).

Table 8.1 Real government expenditure on the personal social services (United Kingdom)

	£m (1987/8 prices)[1]	Year on year % increase	Index of real spending (1973/4 = 100)
1973/4	2,478	–	100
1974/5	2,875	16.0	116
1975/6	3,202	11.4	129
1976/7	3,266	1.9	132
1977/8	2,839	–13.1	115
1978/9	2,922	2.9	118
1979/80	3,132	7.2	126
1980/1	3,304	5.5	133
1981/2	3,266	–1.2	132
1982/3	3,300	1.0	133
1983/4	3,408	3.3	138
1984/5	3,460	1.5	140
1985/6	3,783	9.3	153
1986/7	3,974	5.0	160
1987/8	3,856	–3.0	156
1988/9	4,050	5.0	163
1989/90	4,141	2.2	167
1990/1	4,504	8.8	181
1991/2[2]	4,819	7.0	194

Notes: [1] GDP deflator; [2] 1991/2 = estimated out-turn
Source: Baldock (1994)

Women as workers in the personal social services

Whatever the changes to the organisation, size and scope of the personal social services, there are some continuities in the experiences of women as workers in these services. In systematically considering these experiences there are limited data on which to draw in relation to the workforce of statutory, voluntary and private organisations. There is no comprehensive workforce profile of organisations providing personal social services in Britain.

The only workforce personal social service statistics that are regularly collected relate to the workforce of local authority SSDs. While these are far from detailed with regard to ethnicity, gender, age and disability, they provide some context within which to begin to examine women's experiences as workers in the personal social services. Assumptions based on this limited evidence can be tentatively made about the way in which women are represented in the workforce of the voluntary and private organisations which contribute to the personal social services.

Women form the vast majority of those employed by Social Services Departments (see Table 8.2). Data published in 1990 on England and Wales showed that 86.5 per cent of the workforce in SSDs were women and most of these were employed as part-time workers. The differential distribution of men and women in the SSD workforce

Table 8.2 Staff employed in Social Services Departments in England and Wales in March 1990

	Number	Percentages	Totals (%)
Full-time female	121,320	33.3	86.5 female
Part-time female	193,904	53.2	
Full-time male	43,088	11.8	13.5 male
Part-time male	6,473	1.7	
Totals	364,785	100.0	

Source: LACSAB/ADSS (1990)

is marked. Social Services Departments are pyramid organisations in which women dominate the base and men outnumber women at the peak. This organisational distribution of men and women has not changed significantly since the creation of local authority SSDs in 1971.

Residential care provides one example of this continuity in women's roles as workers. In 1967 the Williams Committee reviewed residential care provision in the personal social services and pointed out that the traditional dependence of this area of the personal social services on women staff (most of whom were single women) had resulted in low pay, low status for care workers and growing staff shortages. The Committee argued that higher status and professional recognition were essential to secure the future of satisfactory residential care services. Over twenty years later the Wagner Committee's review of residential care pointed to the continuing dominance of women in this area of work in local authority, Social Services Departments. They noted:

A commonly held view of care work is that it is unskilled and consists of little more than domestic chores. It is seen as particularly suitable for women, consistent with their traditional roles in the home as carers. A consequence is that the work is seen as less appropriate for men, and there are few male care assistants. Residential work, like other occupations in which women are numerically predominant, is low paid, with low status and poor conditions of service. (Wagner Committee, 1988: 75)

At the top of the local authority pyramid the distribution of men and women also shows a tenaciously consistent pattern over time (see Table 8.3). A more detailed breakdown of the 1990 statistics supplied by different kinds of local authorities Social Services Departments in England and Wales shows little significant difference in the experiences of men and women managers across the range of departments (see Table 8.4). Unfortunately the available local authority SSD statistics tell us little about the diversity of women employed by SSDs with regard to such characteristics as ethnicity, age or disability. However, a recent Department of Health and Social Services Inspectorate study of women in the social services suggest that there are important differences between the experiences of White women workers and women workers from Black and ethnic minorities in the area of the personal social services.

Table 8.3 Percentages of men and women in senior management posts in Social Services Departments in England 1971–90

	1971		1976		1990	
	M	F	M	F	M	F
Director of social services	90	10	91	9	89	11
Deputy director			86	14	90	10
Divisional assistant directors			82	18	80	20

Source: SSI/DoH (1991)

Table 8.4 Senior managers in Social Services Departments in England and Wales 1990

	Directors		Deputies		Assistant divisional directors or equivalent		Totals		%	
	M	F	M	F	M	F	M	F	M	F
English counties	38	1	30	3	185	36	253	40	86	14
English Metropolitan Districts	31	5	24	2	111	26	166	33	83	17
London Boroughs	25	7	12	2	79	34	116	43	73	27
Welsh Authorities	7	1	6	1	29	5	42	7	86	14
Totals	101	14	72	8	404	101	577	123		
Percentages	88	12	90	10	80	20	82	18		

Source: SSI/DoH (1991)

Overall, Black and ethnic minority staff are under-represented in the workforce of local authority SSDs. At the same time

> there tend to be more Afro-Caribbean staff employed in SSDs than other ethnic minority groups. There are hardly any black women at more senior levels in departments and those that are in professional posts are often funded through Section 11 rather than mainstream budgets. They are also less evident among groups of part-time staff than in full-time posts and initiatives to in-crease part-time working are therefore less likely to benefit black and minority ethnic women. (SSI/DoH, 1991: 9)

White, Black and ethnic minority women's experiences as workers in the personal social services are a reflection of the general position of women in the workforce. Women are more likely than men to be in low-paid, low-status jobs within occupations as well as in the labour market generally. At the same time the experiences of White, Black and ethnic minority women differ in relation to part- and full-time work and the opportunities afforded to them within organisations (Abbott and Wallace, 1990).

The world of the local authority personal social services is one in which mainly White, often part-time women workers serve the front line of the service negotiating the distribution of scarce resources (including their own time and skills) in the face of the needs of (predominantly women) service users, while the majority of the full-time White men are employed to supervise and manage resources. The private and voluntary organisations as well as the informal caring which contributes to the personal social services tend to reflect similar patterns. Women mostly in part-time paid capacities as well as full-time unpaid capacities provide the bulk of direct servicing and play a limited role in making decisions about the financing and allocation of resources.

The outcomes of the decisions which are made by predominantly male managers and politicians about resources can be seen in the patterns of differential investments which local authority social services make in services for a range of client groups (see Table 8.5). As women are the main users of personal social services these patterns of investment have a gendered significance. The impact of the distribution of these resources on women's lives has been largely unexplored by central and local government. Official accounts of the personal social services have promoted visions of the relationship between the state, the individual, the family and the community which have been devoid of any explicit consideration of women as service users, paid and unpaid care workers and citizens. It has been feminist analysts of social policy and social work who have explored, critiqued and researched in this area. Their work has raised important questions about women and the personal social services which are explored in the remainder of this chapter.

Official visions and feminist critiques

Official visions of the personal social services will now be considered together with feminist critiques in relation to two eras. The first, 1970–83, was primarily shaped by the Seebohm Report's vision of the personal social services as a state provided Social Services Department response to family need. The second, 1984–94, was a period in which government promoted a vision of the personal social services as a mixed economy of individual, family and community care labour, supported, residually, by a range of formal welfare agencies making provision from the private, voluntary and state welfare sectors.

The personal social services 1970–83

Almost thirty years ago the Seebohm Report, in developing the case for a more unified, state-led approach to the delivery of personal social services, strongly promoted a notion of partnership between the state and families and communities 'in

Table 8.5 Local authority personal social services expenditure England 1984/5: estimated breakdown by client group

	£ thousand	%
Services for elderly people	995,073	38.4
Services for children	493,828	19.0
Services for people with severe learning difficulties	213,168	8.2
Services for people with physical disabilities	110,385	4.3
Services for people with a mental illness	48,193	1.9
Services not allocated to specified client groups	731,483	28.2
Total spending	2,592,130	

Source: Adapted from DHSS (1987)

need' (Seebohm Report, 1968). In opening the debate on the second reading of the Bill which led to the creation of local authority Social Services Departments, the then Secretary of State, Richard Crossman, declared:

> The primary objective of the personal social services we can best describe as strengthening the capacity of the family to care for its members and to supply, as it were, the family's place where necessary; that is, to provide as far as may be social support or if necessary a home for people who cannot look after themselves or . . . be adequately looked after in their family. This is not the only objective of the personal social services. They have an important role to play in community development, for example. But it has been the idea of forming a 'family' service that has inspired the call for a review of the organisation of the service with which the Bill is concerned. (*Hansard*, 1970: col. 1407)

This vision of state-provided personal social services acting both to strengthen the caring capacity of the family and to replace it was devoid of any gendered consideration of what constituted family care. It took for granted, and so reinforced, the notion that women were 'naturally' to be found on both sides of the front line of the personal social services – as service users and service providers. As users, women, who were providing the domestic and emotional servicing of family life, became the prime targets when the family appeared to fail to provide adequate care to its members. At the same time it was primarily women who were recruited to deliver substitutes for family care because they were considered to have the experience and skills suited for this kind of paid employment.

It was this configuration of women's unpaid and paid work in relation to the personal social services that feminist social policy analysts and social work practitioners explored in the 1970s and early 1980s. Their work explicitly identified women's position within the family as critical to an understanding of women and the welfare state (see e.g. Wilson, 1977, 1980; Land, 1983b; Finch and Groves, 1980, 1983; McIntosh, 1981; Ungerson, 1985; Brook and Davis, 1985; Pascall, 1986). Their questioning of the 'naturalness' of this division of family labour raised questions about the part that women were playing in a service which was so closely concerned with supporting a particular view of family life, family duty and family responsibility. Ungerson suggested that in examining this particular arena of social welfare provision it was important to consider the way in which

> two cross-currents, namely the identification of women as the pivotal characters in family life and the preferential allocation of certain social services to men where a woman, is in some sense 'absent', neatly captures two particular features of the personal social services. These services are at an ideological level, a form of social control, and yet, at a material level, an important resource to those in 'need'. (Ungerson, 1985: 187)

The range of contributors to the feminist critique of the official vision of the personal social services in the 1970s and early 1980s illuminated the way in which women were positioned in relation to these two cross-currents. On the one hand, women found their role as prime carers ideologically and personally reinforced by the operation of a personal social services whose workers sought to investigate and assess their performance as adequate mothers, partners and daughters. On the other hand, in the absence of resources on which to draw in order to substitute for their own family labour, poor women had no choice but to turn to the personal social services for help at times of crisis. At the same time the reorganisation of local authority personal social services following the 1970 Local Authority Social Services Act resulted in a further expansion for women of local employment opportunities.

For some feminists it was the potent combination that the personal social services provided of reinforcement of family responsibility, substitution for family work and paid work opportunities for women which demonstrated the complexities and contradictions of the relationship which existed between women and state welfare services. Through contact with the personal social services some women experienced control and curtailment of their lives whilst others experienced the expansion of choice and opportunity. Some women experienced both, either simultaneously or at different times in their lives.

In critically unravelling this relationship the concepts of women's dependency and caring in both private and public domains became a focus of the feminist critique. The personal social services were viewed as a vivid example of the way in which the state controlled women by treating them as dependants within the nuclear family. The dependency which women experienced was reinforced through the caring for other dependants which they undertook. As Pascall expressed it:

> The price for caring is economic dependence. Looking after people is either done for no pay, within the family, or for low pay in the public sector. Social policy's tendency to promote both these arrangements amounts to the exploitation of one kind of dependency to deal with another. (Pascall, 1986: 29)

In contributing to this analysis, Finch and Groves, in their examination of personal social services community care policies for adults with disabilities and older people, highlighted how the policies promoted by such agencies could work to the disadvantage of women in several important respects. Their focus was on community care policies which were reliant on women who were informally caring for other adults in their own homes. These were women who, they argued, were being exploited in providing undervalued and unpaid domestic labour in the community. They were women who were not receiving recognition or assistance from the personal social services. As a result those working to promote community care were failing to consider the equal opportunity issues which such policies raised.

Finch and Groves concluded that subjecting community care policy and provision to equal opportunity audit would raise issues about the need for payment for informal care, increased investment in substitutes for informal care such as residential care and changes to the labour market so that men and women were equally supported in combining care with paid employment. In their view, failure to address these issues would mean that state agencies, such as the personal social services, would continue to subject women, as carers, to unequal treatment in society. As they put it:

> the cultural definition of women as carers is still strong, and since it is part of a set of assumptions about the sexual division of labour in the domestic sphere, it continues to be reinforced and reproduced by a whole range of social and financial policies which unquestionably embody the notion of women's dependency. (Finch and Groves, in Ungerson, 1985: 229)

Feminist critiques of the personal social services in the 1970s and early 1980s illuminated the contradictions and dilemmas of women's experience of state welfare provision. They also highlighted the way in which some women as users and workers were struggling to resolve and move beyond these contradictions (see, for example, the Birmingham Women and Social Work Group, in Brook and Davis, 1985: 115). Yet these critiques were also limited. In particular they took scant account of the diversity of experience amongst women in relation to state-funded welfare services. There was little consideration at this time of the different perspectives and experiences of Black women, women from minority ethnic groups, disabled women and lesbian women in relation to the personal social services.

For Black women the experience of state welfare services had some distinctly different connotations. As Bryan *et al.* describe in their account of the lives of Black women in Britain, 'There is no single area of our lives which better exposes our experience of institutionalised racism than our relationship with the various welfare services' (Bryan *et al.*, 1985: 110). Black women's experiences of the personal social services as citizens, users and workers have demonstrated to them over decades that it has consistently failed to give equal consideration and support to their needs, the ways in which they manage their lives and those dependent on them. In reacting to this lack of formal response some Black women organised themselves through voluntary, private and informal organisations dedicated to delivering services to Black communities as well as campaigning for Black people's rights to local state services (see e.g. Wilson, 1978; Mama, in Walmsley *et al.*, 1993: 96). As a result they were positioned differently from White women in areas of the voluntary, informal and private areas of the personal social services as well as in the state services.

The personal social services 1984–94

These themes of the commonality and diversity in women's experience of the personal social services were increasingly identified and explored in the social policy and social work feminist literature of the late 1980s and early 1990s (see e.g. Hanmer and Statham, 1988; Dominelli and McLeod, 1989; Hallet, 1989; Maclean and Groves, 1991; Langan and Day, 1992). At the same time the official vision of the kind of personal social services which was fit for this era began to shift radically. This transformation has been described by Baldock and others as a move from a conception of the personal social services as a potentially universalist fifth-state social service responding to individual, family and community need to that of a residual service stepping in when all else failed, a service whose role had to move from being one of main resource provider to that of enabler of other providers in a world where 'the reality is that most care is provided by family, friends and neighbours' (Griffiths, 1988: para. 2.3).

This change was not just directed at the personal social services. It was part of a larger transformation which affected state welfare provision in the decade of the 1980s and 1990s, a transformation which has been described by several authors (McCarthy, 1989; Johnson, 1990; Langan and Clarke, 1994) as being characterised by a concern to bring market forces to bear on the delivery and management of state welfare. Thus the notion of the state taking responsibility for delivering services to strengthen family and community through local authority Social Services Departments gave way to a vision of the state withdrawing from direct service provision in order to stimulate and enable a mixed economy response to those assessed as in need of the personal social services. This shift was heralded in several speeches from government ministers, several government reports (e.g. Audit Commission, 1986; Griffiths Report, 1988) and found legal expression in two major pieces of personal social service legislation, the Children Act 1989 and the National Health Service and Community Care Act 1990.

In 1984 Norman Fowler, then Minister of Social Security, addressing the Annual Joint Conference of Directors of Social Services, officially launched the notion that the personal social services should not encourage dependence on the state. Instead self-reliance should be promoted through Social Services Departments working 'to enable the greatest possible number of individuals to act reciprocally, giving and receiving services for the well-being of the whole community' (Fowler, 1984, quoted in McCarthy, 1989: 25). Two years later this vision was elaborated as Fowler rejected the notion that the state should take responsibility for providing care in the community and suggested that a more efficient use of resources would result from stimulating a mixed economy of personal social services provision (Fowler, 1986). As feminist critiques demonstrated, this vision could only be sustained by women, who, as individual family members, friends and good neighbours, were providing care in an unpaid capacity, and who, as part-time low-paid care workers, were providing labour for the private, voluntary and the (diminishing) state sectors of the personal social services. But there was no explicit acknowledgement by government of the role which they assumed women would play in delivering the vision. The language used was ungendered. Service users, providers and purchasers were the main players in a world where choice, flexibility and a more personalised response to need were the promised outcomes. Gender, social division, unemployment and increasing poverty were not part of the context of change.

As several commentators have pointed out, however, this vision of the personal social services owed much to the efforts of a government trying to manage an economy in which a growing number of poor people of all ages as well as a growing number of older people were turning for assistance to the personal social services (Harding, 1992; Schorr, 1992; Clarke *et al.*, 1994) and a government struggling to curb public expenditure through curtailing local authority power and the resources available for personal social services provision. It was in this context that the two major pieces of legislation which are currently shaping priorities in the personal social services should be understood. The Children Act 1989 established a framework for providing services for children 'in need' and families in a manner which Langan has described as involving

> a voluntary partnership between the family and the state in which the family acts as a consumer of a range of services, such as accommodation, day care and social work support. In the spirit of the new mixed economy of welfare these services are to be provided either directly by the state, or preferably by other agencies coordinated by the social services department. (Langan, in Clarke, 1993: 156)

The National Health Service and Community Care Act 1990 established a minimalist approach in which local authorities were given a remit to allocate scarce resources on the basis of needs assessment of adults requiring care in the community. Both Acts drew on ungendered accounts of family relationships reflecting none of the burgeoning evidence of the changes taking place in British society in respect to women's roles, family values and diversifying family forms (Finch, 1990; Baldock and Ungerson, 1993; Finch and Mason, 1993).

In response to these omissions feminist critiques have looked explicitly at the way in which women were faring in the shifting terrain of the personal social services. The increasing poverty being experienced by British society as service users has been shown to be falling increasingly on women as parents, disabled people and older people (Glendinning and Millar, 1992; Oppenheim, 1993). Such women were finding the gap widening between the resources they had to manage on and what they had to manage in their households and communities. One consequence was that 'too many people with too great needs are being directed towards the personal social services'

(Schorr, 1992: 48). The resultant strain was falling on women as the majority of service users and front-line workers.

Front-line personal social service staff are increasingly faced with difficult, if not impossible, caring and emotional work. Rather than operating to increase women's choice and opportunity, services have in fact been increasingly driven by a rationed response to crisis. This is not, of course, just happening in local authority Social Services Departments. As a consequence of stimulating a mixed economy of provision women have been experiencing change in the location of their employment within the personal social services. With the increasing use of 'contracted-out' services the pattern has emerged of a core, professional and highly paid staff within the state sector and a growing peripheral, short-term, poorly paid staff in the mix of private, voluntary and state agencies. As Newman has observed, it is at the periphery that women increasingly find themselves:

> The effects are experienced most acutely by black women who form the backbone of many of the contracted-out services in the cleaning, catering and laundry services. Women in the contracted-out services have tended to lose their security of employment and the benefits however slight of working for a good employment. . . . For black and white women in the 'flexible' arm of the organisational labour force, then, things are getting worse. (Newman, 1994: 188)

The issues of women's dependence, their role *vis-à-vis* the family and their caring labour still hold the key to understanding the impact on women which legislative, managerial and political change are currently having on the personal social services. Feminist analysts in this period have suggested that these issues now need to be understood in a context in which the role of the state has shifted in respect of both employment and service delivery in the personal social services.

Conclusion

In reviewing the personal social services in the United Kingdom in the early 1990s Alvin Schorr (formerly an American adviser to the Seebohm Committee in the 1960s) noted several features which suggest that increasingly residual, means-tested, fragmented and disorganised services are being offered to poor people. It is a view which contrasts markedly with the managerial language of market-led, efficient and effective responses to need which mark the official visions of the personal social services. It is within this gap between official rhetoric and an increasingly difficult reality that women as citizens, service users and workers are having to negotiate the transformation of the personal social services.

9   *Women and community care*

Susan Tester

Community care embraces many of the social policy areas covered in previous chapters and forms a large component of the UK government's policy on caring for adults with long-term care needs. Reforms implemented in the early 1990s introduced changes to the systems of funding and providing community care and incorporated expectations about the roles and responsibilities of informal carers. Community care has particular salience for women since the majority of these informal carers and the majority of people with care needs are women.

This chapter explores the issues surrounding the provision and receipt of community care, drawing mainly on literature and experiences from the United Kingdom, supplemented by references to trends elsewhere in Europe. First, definitions of community care are considered and developments in community care policies in the United Kingdom and Europe are traced. The chapter then focuses on community care as an issue for women and on the implications for women's lives of informal and formal care in the context of reformed systems and shifts in the welfare mix. Finally, the future of care based on the family model is discussed.

Approaches to the definition of community care

Defining 'community care' is no simple matter since meanings of the concept are both vague and shifting. The term, evoking, as Titmuss (1968: 104) suggested, 'a sense of

warmth and human kindness, essentially personal and comforting', has proved inval-
uable for political rhetoric. It can conveniently be adapted to loosely defined policy
goals with which few politicians or voters could disagree. The rhetoric, however,
masks a reality which is often disadvantageous to women, entailing unpaid care given
or received with little support from formal services.

The 'community' component of the concept is arguably the source of much ambiguity, and is rarely used in this way in other languages (Jamieson, 1989). 'Community' has diverse meanings, mostly with desirable connotations at a rhetorical level.
Where women are concerned, 'community' may be used positively to mean women's
space, where they can organise together outside the home to improve living conditions; but when used in the term 'community care' its meaning is the more restrictive
one of women's *place*, where women take on the responsibilities of unpaid care in the
home (Williams, 1993: 33–4). The use of 'community' to describe the location and/or
source of care is misleading. As a location for care 'community' is used to contrast
with 'institution', yet, as Higgins (1989: 5–7) points out, the distinction between the
two is not clear-cut. Some community care, such as day and respite care, can be
offered in institutions, and some institutional care, such as group homes or hostels,
can be provided in the community. 'Community' as a source of care is a myth since,
as many writers have stressed, in practice most care is provided by the family, mainly
by female relatives (see e.g. Finch and Groves, 1980, 1983).

The 'care' component of the concept also entails lack of clarity as it covers a wide
range of caring tasks and of housing, health and welfare services to support people
with long-term care needs. However, in much of the UK feminist literature, 'caring'
is perceived as informal care given in the home by (informal) 'carers' to adults with
care needs, although, as Ungerson (1990) points out, these are very limited meanings
compared with those used in Scandinavian countries to cover all types of care for
children and adults.

Community care policies originated in moves against care in large, often remote
institutions such as hospitals and residential homes for people with mental and
physical illnesses and disabilities. The main rationales for such moves were, first, that
institutional care was considered by politicians to be too expensive and, second, that
such care was undesirable for the individuals concerned, as found by writers such as
Goffman (1961) and Townsend (1962). The changing emphases on the 'organisational' and 'humanitarian' reasons for community care policies (Macintyre, 1977) and
the potential conflicts between them are further sources of ambiguity in the meaning
of community care.

Early community care policies in the United Kingdom, then, envisaged such care
in contrast to the institutionalisation of adults with long-term care needs. Care was to
be provided in the community by professionals and agencies for people living in
ordinary housing, for example by domiciliary and day care services, or in specialised
settings such as hostels, group homes or sheltered housing. The emphasis in the
1960s was on humanitarian principles and the provision, mainly by statutory agencies, of services in community-based settings, which were considered preferable to
large institutions. By the late 1970s, however, policy makers, influenced by economic

crises and demographic projections of rapidly increasing numbers of very elderly people, perceived such care provision as too expensive and the emphasis moved to economic concerns and cost containment.

Such considerations promoted a key shift in the concept of community care from care *in* the community to care *by* the community, as stated, for example in the White Paper *Growing Older* (DHSS, 1981a: 3), which also held that 'the primary sources of support and care for elderly people are informal and voluntary. These spring from the personal ties of kinship, friendship and neighbourhood.' The role of public authorities was defined as that of sustaining and developing such care, since, as also stated in *Care in Action* (DHSS, 1981b: 32), 'Public authorities will not command the resources to deal with it alone.' The community was thus perceived as an inexpensive and humanitarian source of care for dependent adults. As suggested above, however, the reality of the community as a source of care means that the majority of care is provided by women. This shift in the meaning of community care prompted a decade of feminist critiques of community care policies (Finch, 1990).

Changes and lack of clarity in definitions of community care mean that this term has little value. It embraces the whole gamut of long-term care provision for people who live in their own homes, which may be in ordinary housing or carers' homes, specialised or residential settings. For the purposes of policy analysis and of identifying implications for women, it is therefore useful to divide the concept into basic components: the caring tasks or services offered, the settings in which care is provided, the care providers and the financers of care (Tester, 1995). The tasks and services include housing and financial support as well as basic help with daily living and self-care activities, medical, nursing and rehabilitation services, emotional support for carers and cared-for, social and leisure activities, transport and information. The care may be provided in the home, for example domiciliary care, or the person may travel to another venue such as a clinic or day centre to receive care.

In practice most community care is provided by the informal sector (family, friends and neighbours). Formal care is offered by statutory authorities, voluntary non-profit-making organisations and commercial agencies. Distinctions between formal and informal care and their implications for women are discussed further below. Care is financed mainly by the individual with care needs, the family, the state, insurance funds and charities. Trends in social policy and in community care since the late 1970s led to shifts in the balance between the different care providers and funders in the mixed economy of welfare (Evers and Svetlik, 1993).

Development of community care policies in the United Kingdom and Europe

Official reports and policy documents in the 1980s showed that community care, although a policy goal for several decades, had not been implemented successfully in the United Kingdom (House of Commons, 1985; Audit Commission, 1986; Griffiths

Report, 1988). Problems identified included low standards, inequitable distribution of services, poor management, inefficiency, lack of co-ordination, and 'perverse incentives' in the social security system which encouraged residential care in private and voluntary sector homes through income support payments. The White Paper *Caring for People* (HMSO, 1989, Cmnd 849) incorporated many of Griffiths' recommendations and the National Health Service and Community Care Act 1990 legislated for changes to the systems of funding and delivering community care, implemented from 1991 to 1993 (see Meredith, 1995).

The economic, demographic and political factors which prompted the United Kingdom's community care reforms were also influential in other European countries during the 1980s, as similar reports and reviews of systems were published and reforms were initiated (Jamieson, 1991; Baldock and Evers, 1992; Walker *et al.*, 1993; Tester, 1995). The main changes to the UK system are outlined below in the context of wider European trends.

From the late 1970s and throughout the 1980s and early 1990s economic concerns were predominant and cost containment and cost effectiveness became major policy goals for European governments. The UK reforms thus aimed to remove the perverse incentives in the social security system and to 'secure better value for taxpayers' money' (HMSO, 1989: 5) through a new funding system giving local authorities responsibility for assessing needs and purchasing residential or community-based care for people requiring state financial assistance. This system entailed increased targeting of services to people with highest-priority needs and rationing of services through stricter criteria and/or increased charges to users. Changes to funding systems for long-term care were similarly proposed or implemented in the early 1990s in other European countries (Laing, 1993a).

Another aspect of the concern for cost containment was a trend towards reducing institutional care because community care was considered to be less expensive, although such calculations rarely take account of unpaid informal care, as discussed further below. The UK reforms aimed 'to promote the development of domiciliary, day and respite services' (HMSO, 1989: 5), so that people with care needs could remain in their own homes rather than enter institutional care. The new funding system only supported in residential care people with low incomes assessed as needing such care. In the Netherlands the policy of 'substitution' similarly promoted the use of community-based, social or informal care rather than institutional, technical or professional care (Tunissen and Knapen, 1991; Baldock and Evers, 1992). The aim of reducing institutional care was common to most north-western European countries, for example Denmark and Germany.

Reduction of public expenditure was an ideological as well as an economic goal, espoused by politicians of the New Right such as Margaret Thatcher, who also sought to lower taxation, to decrease the state's role in direct provision of housing, health and welfare services, and to encourage individual and family responsibility. Such views promoted the trend towards developing the role of non-statutory sectors in the mixed economy of welfare, entailing increased use of the private and informal sectors of care provision and the stimulation of markets and competition in care services. In the

United Kingdom, where the state was a major provider of care services, under the reformed community care system local authorities were expected to make increased use of voluntary and commercial sector providers whose services were purchased under contracting arrangements. The development of innovative forms of provision with different service providers and localised services was part of this trend in different areas of Europe (Kraan *et al.*, 1991; Nijkamp *et al.*, 1991; Evers and van der Zanden, 1993).

Policy makers also began to recognise more explicitly the major role which informal carers had always played in care provision. In the United Kingdom feminist critiques of community care contributed to placing the issue of carers on the policy agenda and to the inclusion in government policy of the objective 'to ensure that service providers make practical support for carers a high priority' (HMSO, 1989: 5). The importance of supporting carers in continuing to provide unpaid care in the home was also recognised in, for example, France (Boulard, 1991; Schopflin, 1991).

Linked to this recognition of carers as valuable sources of unpaid care were more humanitarian moves towards providing flexible care tailored to the needs of individuals and their carers, rather than offering standard services, as advocated, for example in policies in the United Kingdom (HMSO, 1989) and the Netherlands (Dekker Committee, 1987). The United Kingdom's reforms introduced a system of assessment and care management whereby local authorities were responsible for assessing individual needs and arranging 'packages of care', taking account of users' and carers' preferences. The local authorities' increased responsibilities for overall planning, for individual assessment and for purchasing services were also intended to address the difficulties of co-ordination between services which had led to gaps and overlaps in services to individuals. Similarly, housing, social and health care services for older people in Sweden were re-organised in 1992, giving responsibility to municipalities (Johannson, 1993).

Economic, demographic, political and ideological influences since the late 1970s thus led to changes in community care delivery and funding systems in the early 1990s. In the context of these trends and policy developments, community care was taken up as a feminist issue in the United Kingdom.

Community care as an issue for women

Feminist social policy writers such as Pascall (1986) and Williams (1989) stress that until the late 1970s and early 1980s women were invisible in mainstream social policy analysis. Similarly, caring work was invisible in community care policy. Caring became one of the main issues on which feminist analysts focused in making women's issues more manifest in social policy. This emphasis continued as feminists responded to the trends in community care outlined above.

Feminist critiques of social policy stress the centrality of understanding the position of women in relation to state welfare, although feminist perspectives differ in their interpretation of this relationship. Whereas mainstream British social policy focused on state-provided welfare, feminist analysts emphasise the role of the family in welfare, the position of women within the family, assumptions about women's caring roles, and women's position as main providers and receivers of welfare services. Such analyses show that British welfare state services since the 1940s, based on the nuclear family with a male breadwinner and a housewife at home, ensured the dependence of married women on their husbands for financial support and for access to state benefits (Pascall, 1986).

In the nuclear family thus favoured by the state it was considered 'natural' for women to undertake caring work for children and for adults with disabilities. Conceptions of caring work as natural for women originate both in patriarchal assumptions and in divisions of labour between men and women in the public and private spheres, arising partly from industrialisation and the operation of capitalist systems. Such systems, reinforced by state welfare support for the nuclear family, depend on social reproduction work carried out in the home, the private sphere, by women to support the male breadwinner/producer in the public sphere (Williams, 1989).

The types of work undertaken by many women within and outside the home tend to consist of providing care and services for family members or other people: as unpaid carers at home, or in welfare or service occupations outside the home, often of lower status than work traditionally carried out by men. Women's earnings power is limited by low pay and the need to take part-time work to fit in with responsibilities at home. Most women, then, cannot afford to pay for care for their relatives, and thus become financially dependent through providing unpaid care at home themselves (Graham, 1993a).

Feminist writers draw attention to the exploitation of women in unpaid or low-paid caring work, as discussed further below, while also emphasising that many women's identity is derived from their caring roles and relationships. Graham (1983), for example, argues that the 'labour' and 'love' components of caring should be analysed together by the discipline of social policy, which had concentrated on the labour aspects, whereas psychology had examined the emotional aspects of caring and neglected the work and stress involved. Women's caring work can thus be analysed according to divisions of labour between men and women, between the private and public spheres and according to different aspects of the caring role.

Feminists stress that state welfare policies to support the family promoted the nuclear family model (Pascall, 1986: 38). Dalley (1988: 20) maintains that the dominant ideology of familism 'operates as a principle of social organisation at both the domestic and public level, especially in the field of social care'. This ideology assumes that women will undertake caring work: an assumption rarely acknowledged in state policy until community care policies in the 1980s made explicit expectations that the family (mainly women) would provide most caring services at home, with the state taking a residual role. Such expectations continued to be based on the assumption that women will be at home to provide care; in spite of women's increased participation in the paid workforce, 'it is still portrayed as natural to care and unnatural not to do so' (Brown and Smith, 1993: 187).

The reasons why women are expected to be available and willing to provide care are explored by feminists. Ungerson finds that carers are selected 'according to dominant, normative, and gendered rules of kinship' (1987: 61), then by negotiation with other members of the family. Research suggests a basic hierarchy of caring responsibilities for older people with first preference to a spouse, then to a daughter, a daughter-in-law, a son, then another relative or non-relative (Qureshi and Walker, 1989). Further factors, such as employment status, stage in the life cycle, beliefs and value systems, enter into the process of negotiation as to which individual family members take on the main caring role (Ungerson, 1987; Finch, 1989). Finch and Mason argue that 'Responsibilities are *created* rather than flowing automatically from specific relationships' (1993: 167). Women are more likely than men to be under pressure to take on caring and, if necessary, to give up paid work, particularly if they are in low-paid jobs. Women, then, are expected to undertake caring for family members with long-term care needs even when there are competing demands of paid work and/or child care: a requirement described as 'compulsory altruism' (Land and Rose, 1985).

Caring undertaken within the family or in family-like settings is often perceived as based on the motherhood model, appropriate to the tending of children, but not necessarily to the care of dependent adults (Ungerson, 1983). The motherhood model entails infantilisation of adults with disabilities and an emphasis on bodily needs and physical dependence rather than on social and emotional needs (Hockey and James, 1993). Such infantilisation affects the relationship between carer and cared-for and may be difficult to accept by those who have previously had a more equal relationship, or when the roles or balance of power between, for example a mother and daughter, have been reversed (Ungerson, 1983; Lewis and Meredith, 1988).

Feminist critiques of community care in the 1990s

Feminist critiques in the 1980s were mainly advanced from the perspective of younger, female, non-disabled carers and neglected the older female recipients of care and the caring roles of older and disabled women (Graham, 1993a). In the 1990s feminists with disabilities, such as Begum (1990) and Morris (1991–2), drew attention to this one-dimensional analysis and focused on the experiences of women with disabilities and the implications for them of community care. Morris points out that feminists' emphasis on the burden of caring meant that those cared for were perceived mainly as dependent objects of care. She suggests that a more appropriate focus for research would be the caring relationship, bridging distinctions between carer and cared-for (Morris, 1991–2).

It is clearly important to examine the complex issues of dependence and independence for both parties in a caring relationship. Care-givers are often economically dependent on male partners or the state. People cared for in the community are frequently considered to be living independently in their own homes, but may in fact be dependent for basic needs on a relative (Williams, 1989: 195). There are normative expectations of carers and recipients of care which cannot always be met. Aronson's research showed that older women who needed care tried to maintain their self-esteem and independence by limiting their demands on carers, whereas younger women tried in their own interests to set limits on care-giving. Both groups thus attempted to manage the tensions between ideology and the reality of their situation (Aronson, 1990).

Feminists highlighted gender differences in expectations about the caring tasks to be carried out, with an emphasis on women's role in physical care, including mothering skills and the management of incontinence (Ungerson, 1983). Research focusing on caring daughters, however, neglected the substantial role of men in caring for spouses and partners, particularly in the older age groups (Arber and Ginn, 1990). Younger women with disabilities may be cared for by male partners and resent assumptions that men will not undertake caring roles (Morris, 1991–2: 37). Women with disabilities are also expected to accept the consequences of disability, such as dependence and loss of paid employment, more readily than men (Brown and Smith, 1993: 191).

Experiences and expectations of community care, dependence and independence differ not only by gender and disability but also by social class, age, 'race' and sexual preference. The need for informal care varies by social class. Those in lower social classes are more likely than others to experience poor health and disability, but less likely to have financial and other resources to gain access to formal care (Arber and Ginn, 1992) and less likely to have access to informal care and family support (Graham, 1993a: 130). Among informal carers there are social class differences in provision of co-resident care, the most demanding form of care; of men and women carers under 45 those in the lowest social classes are most likely to be co-resident carers (Arber and Ginn, 1992: 627). There are also age differences in that middle-class people are more likely to need care at an older age than working-class people, and that men are more likely to provide co-resident care in the older age groups, whereas women's responsibility for such care peaks in middle age (45–64) (Arber and Ginn, 1992: 625).

Community care policy expectations about family care, based on the White British family and British values, are often inappropriate to minority ethnic communities from widely different cultures and with varying family patterns. Further, service providers tend to stereotype Black people as living in extended families which care for their members, a model which still applies to some Asian families but rarely to other groups. Assumptions are then made that Black families and carers do not need support from formal services (Walker and Ahmad, 1994). In practice immigration controls and employment patterns have restricted opportunities for Black people to live with their families and care for each other. The experience of Black women employed in caring for other people's families in domestic or health care settings has been neglected by feminist studies on caring (Graham, 1991: 69, 1993a: 128–9).

Similarly, little research has been undertaken on the community care experiences of lesbians. Care services are based on familist norms that promote the heterosexual nuclear family and stigmatise other family forms and living arrangements (Stacey, 1991). Older or disabled lesbians are among those women who will not necessarily have family carers such as daughters, but may have partners or other adult support networks. Working-class and/or Black lesbians dependent on low-paid employment or state pensions and benefits have restricted access to financial resources and private caring options. However, lesbians' specific needs for formal services are often 'unrecognised and ignored' (Brown, 1992).

Critiques of community care in the 1990s thus highlight the need to recognise inequalities between women and examine interactions of class, age, 'race', disability and sexual preference which may compound disadvantages and lead to differences in experiences of giving and receiving care.

Implications of community care for women's lives

The development of feminist critiques revealed multiple dimensions of community care to be taken into account in a more comprehensive analysis than those of the 1980s. Implications of community care for women's lives are examined below with reference to relevant social divisions and to the relations between different types and locations of care.

Distinctions between formal and informal, public and private were used in the 1980s for analysis of the divisions of labour between state and family and between men and women in the public and private domains, and for making visible women's unpaid caring work. Feminists in the 1990s, however, criticised the earlier acceptance of policy makers' assumptions that caring is mainly undertaken by female relatives in the home (Aronson, 1990; Ungerson, 1990; Graham, 1991). This acceptance meant that the public/private division of caring work was not questioned, and that the ways in which the labour and love aspects of women's caring work span both spheres were not examined. Ungerson suggests that, rather than using a 'false dichotomy' between public and private, 'it might be more illuminating to consider the two contexts of care together and understand their similarities and differences by analysing them together' (1990: 12). Graham identifies the need to distinguish 'between the location and social relations of care' rather than assuming that care at home means care by family, and excluding other types of care in the home (1991: 65). She argues that this association of the home with family care has focused on middle-class women's experience of the private domain, to which working-class or Black women have less access (Graham, 1991: 69, 73). The emphasis in feminist perspectives thus shifted in the 1990s to the importance of perceiving and analysing caring work across the public/private divide.

The relationship between formal and informal care also received attention in the context of reforms to the United Kingdom's community care systems implemented in the early 1990s, as outlined above. Trends such as the pursuit of cost effectiveness, the reduction in institutional care, and the development of the non-statutory sectors of the welfare mix placed greater emphasis on informal care. This meant that women were increasingly likely to give or receive such care. Policy makers were also aware of the need for services to support carers in continuing to provide unpaid care, and promoted the design of individual packages of care based on assessed needs of users and carers (HMSO, 1989). In practice, however, there was little development of effective support for carers; such support cost the formal sector very little and carers were seen mainly as a 'resource whose "price" to social care agencies was very low' (Twigg and Atkin, 1993: 6).

The relationship between carers and service providers involved in such arrangements has received little attention in policy analysis. Twigg and Atkin (1993: 11–15) propose four models. First, carers are seen as 'resources' providing free services; there is an implicit assumption that carers, if available, will give such care. Second, carers are perceived as 'co-workers' with the formal agencies. Third, the most heavily burdened carers are considered as 'co-clients' needing help to cope with their situation. The fourth category is the 'superseded carer'; the agency either helps the disabled person to become independent of the carer, or supports the carer in giving up caring responsibilities. It is likely that in most cases the carer is the prime service provider and that formal services are only offered when the carer is unable to care alone or needs support to continue to do so. In effect the principle of subsidiarity is applied, although not explicitly, as in Germany, where family members are required, in certain situations, to provide care (Tester, 1994).

The costs to the carer are usually omitted from the equation in policy statements advocating community care as 'cheaper' than institutional care or substituting less formal types of provision. Such costs are, however, recognised in the United Kingdom in a substantial body of qualitative and quantitative research, including that commissioned by the government, conducted since the late 1970s (summarised by Parker, 1990; Twigg, 1992). This research includes feminist accounts of caring and a national survey of a representative sample from the 1985 General Household Survey (Green, 1988), data from which have been further analysed by, for example, Arber and Ginn (1990, 1992) and Parker and Lawton (1990).

Such research on informal care describes different groups of carers and people cared for, and the work undertaken by carers. While the satisfaction derived from the caring role is recognised, the main focus is on the burdens entailed. The research highlights physical, emotional, social and financial costs to carers, for example the physical effort of lifting, bathing and toileting those cared for; the 24-hour responsibility and stress; the loss of social contacts, employment opportunities and pension rights (see e.g. Nissel and Bonnerjea, 1982; Finch and Groves, 1983; Lewis and Meredith, 1988; Levin *et al.*, 1989; Qureshi and Walker, 1989; Glendinning, 1992; and, for a European perspective, Jani-Le Bris, 1993).

Such research means that the need to support carers in their role is recognised, whereas before the 1980s their caring work was taken for granted. It has, however, been criticised for stressing the burdens on carers and the dependence of those cared for. It is argued that 'this is not how many carers perceive their situation, and that the language is pathologizing' (Twigg and Atkin, 1993: 5). As discussed earlier, the emphasis moved in the 1990s to analysing the differences of experience between carers (Atkin, 1992) and examining the experiences of people receiving care, which may also be a combination of the positive and the negative (Aronson, 1990).

Physical, emotional, social and financial costs are experienced by those with care needs as well as by carers, although these costs have received less attention. People with disabilities often have difficulties managing activities of daily living and adopt various strategies to continue with such activities before turning to informal or formal care (Wilson, 1994: 239–40). This important contribution of self-care is rarely recognised in policy statements or literature on caring. Lack or loss of personal autonomy has an impact on disabled people's self-esteem and on their relationships (Aronson, 1990). As Morris (1991–2: 35) points out: 'it is the loss of reciprocity which brings about inequality within a relationship'; further, physical, emotional and financial abuse can occur in such unequal relationships. People with care needs have limited access to social, leisure and employment opportunities. They also have financial costs associated with disabilities, and are likely to have limited financial resources and/or to depend on state benefits.

In caring relationships and in decisions about formal support services there are potential conflicts of interest between people with care needs and their carers. There are few choices for either party when unhappy with their situation because alternative sources of care are rarely available (Aronson, 1990). Family care does not always provide a beneficial environment and some people would prefer professional care (Brown and Smith, 1993). Although the rhetoric of community care reforms in the United Kingdom promotes increased user and carer participation and choice, people with disabilities and carers are unlikely to be able to exercise such choice in practice (Walker, 1993).

Community care services in the 1990s

Most care for people with disabilities and illnesses takes the form of self-care or informal care. To support people with care needs and their carers services are offered by formal agencies. Some services are specifically for carers, for example support groups, while others provided for the person cared for, such as day or respite care, also help the carer; decisions on such service provision may involve a conflict of interests between carer and cared-for. The main health and social welfare services offered in the home or other locations are considered further below. Other services, such as housing, social security, leisure and transport, are also crucial to people's ability to live in their own homes. Issues concerning women and a range of services are discussed in previous chapters.

Under the British community care system the local authority's social services/ social work department is responsible for assessing individual needs and arranging a package of care services. To gain access to such services the person with care needs or the carer applies or is referred for entry to the assessment process. Any care package provided is based on informal care networks available (Wenger, 1994). Services may be purchased by the authority from statutory, voluntary and commercial agencies or through innovative arrangements such as payments to neighbours, friends or volunteers to provide specific services (Leat, 1992).

The lives of those involved, the majority of whom are women, are clearly affected by whether or not support services are offered. Access to support from social care services including home care, residential, respite and day care services, is limited under the British system through needs assessment and through financial assessment for contribution to the costs of care. Most services from the National Health Service, however, including long-stay care, hospital treatment and primary care, although also rationed, are free of charge to the user. People with financial resources or private health insurance are able to purchase services in private health or social care markets without going through assessment systems. Financial help for people with disabilities, for example disability living allowance and attendance allowance, or for carers, for example invalid care allowance, is subject to strict criteria and makes only a limited contribution to the actual costs involved. Charities provide some assistance with care costs but have limited resources in the context of increasing demands.

Socio-economic class is clearly an important determinant of the choices people have in care services, as those in the higher classes often have greater financial resources, knowledge of the systems and skills to negotiate access to them. People most likely to need services, however, such as women in the oldest age groups and those from minority ethnic groups and their carers, are least likely to have information about services (Tester, 1992).

Access to appropriate services is also affected by household composition, gender, age, 'race' and sexual preference. Domiciliary services are mainly provided to people living alone, rarely to those with co-resident carers; carers aged over 65 are more likely to receive support than younger ones (Arber et al., 1988). Women with disabilities are less likely than men to receive help with domestic tasks because of assumptions about the division of labour in the home (Arber and Ginn, 1991: 147); people from minority ethnic groups tend to underuse formal services. Provision of care services for Black people is criticised as inappropriate to their needs. It is not merely a question of taking account of special needs, a process which can marginalise users, but also of addressing structural inequalities in the systems of provision (Atkin, 1991; Walker and Ahmad, 1994). Similarly, it is argued that the needs and preferences of lesbians, for example for bereavement counselling, support services or residential care, should be met, but that attention should also be paid to non-discriminatory practice (Brown, 1992).

The policy rhetoric of the United Kingdom's community care reforms advocates humanitarian goals such as packages of care which would meet individual needs more appropriately. Systems of assessment and care management, however, are in the early stages of implementation and progress is uneven across the country (Baldock and Ungerson, 1993; Department of Health, 1994b; Warner, 1994). The economic goals of cost containment conflict with the aims of providing appropriate services to users and carers. Cash-limited budgets are targeted to highest-priority needs, which tend to be for nursing or residential home care. There are unresolved issues of division of responsibilities between health and social services in the context of reductions in NHS long-stay beds; the health and social care systems were not integrated by the reforms to the organisation and funding of community care. In these circumstances lower-priority needs are unlikely to be met, services such as home care are reduced or withdrawn, and charges to users are increased (Age Concern England, 1993; Warner, 1994).

The reformed system entails a shift to greater use of non-statutory sectors in the welfare mix, either through purchase of services by local authorities or because people turn to these sectors for care which cannot be provided by local government. This shift to a market system of care purchased from voluntary and private sectors disadvantages Black and minority ethnic groups, whose own voluntary service-providing organisations may find it difficult to compete for contracts (Atkin, 1991). The shift in the welfare mix has implications for women as carers and cared-for. Greater demands are made on informal carers when high levels of care needs cannot be met by formal services. As paid care work is transferred to the private and voluntary sectors and to volunteers or neighbours who work for token payments, pay and working conditions, as well as standards of service, may be unsatisfactory and difficult to regulate (Brown and Smith, 1993; Walker, 1993). Trends in the mixed economy of welfare thus work to the disadvantage of many women across social divisions and the boundaries of types and locations of care.

Conclusion: women and community care in the future

The concept 'community care' as used in the United Kingdom covers a wide range of caring tasks and services for adults with physical and mental disabilities and illnesses. Care is given by unpaid carers and paid workers, the majority of whom are women, in the home or in settings outside the home, in a mixed economy of welfare provision and funding comprising informal, statutory, non-profit and commercial sectors. Reformed systems in the United Kingdom and elsewhere in Europe have shifted the balance of the welfare mix away from statutory and formal services. This chapter raises many of the issues concerning the division of caring work between men and women and across the public and private domains in the context of changing systems and political and economic conditions.

The role of women as the main providers of informal care was placed on the agenda by feminist critiques in the 1980s, focusing on community care as an aspect of social policy which illustrated wider issues concerning the role of the nuclear family in state welfare, the division of labour between men and women, and assumptions that caring was women's 'natural' role. Feminist social policy analysts considered alternative forms of care, and concluded that non-sexist forms of community care were unlikely to be developed, and that forms of residential care based on collectivism rather than familism would be more appropriate solutions (Finch, 1984; Dalley, 1988).

Feminists in the 1990s take a wider perspective than that of the able-bodied younger female carer; they examine not only gender differences in caring but also experiences of women of different social class, age, 'race', disability and sexual prefer-ence. Such perspectives bridge unhelpful distinctions between carer and cared-for, formal and informal, public and private, dependence and independence in analysing women's experiences of giving and receiving care. Their solutions for the future give consideration to the views of people with care needs and their individual preferences for residential or family-based care or innovative forms of living arrangements, and the types of care and support to be offered in public and private domains (Finch, 1990; Ungerson, 1990; Morris, 1991–2).

Critiques of the United Kingdom's reformed community care system show that the problems identified in the 1980s by government reports and by feminists have not yet been resolved. Although the reformed system has the potential to provide appro-priate services to meet the needs and preferences of users and carers, in practice the main thrust of the reforms has been containment of the costs of institutional care. The system continues to assume that the family, mainly women, will provide most of the care and to shift a higher level of responsibilities to the informal sector. Women are also exploited as low-paid workers in an increasingly fragmented system. In spite of gestures toward involving users and carers in service planning and individual assessment, the system perpetuates inequalities among women according to social class, 'race' and other social divisions.

The model of the White, heterosexual, nuclear family on which community care is based rests on outdated assumptions. In the late twentieth century the decline in full employment for men, the increase in women's paid work, and rising numbers of one-parent families and other family forms mean that many households no longer depend on the earnings of a male breadwinner. Such changes in demographic and employ-ment patterns have not altered the perception that middle-aged women are the natural carers, and that the decrease in numbers of this age group in relation to increasing proportions in the oldest age groups is a cause for concern across the European Union (Alber, 1993). Difficulties in recruiting paid care workers, for ex-ample in Germany and the Netherlands, have implications for women from disadvan-taged areas such as eastern Europe who may be employed as cheap labour.

Issues in community care to promote the varying interests of women include not only seeking specific improvements to services and support, but longer-term consid-erations of changes to the division of labour between women and men (Finch, 1990: 52–3). Such changes must be seen in the context of worldwide employment patterns and of employment policies in the United Kingdom and Europe (Twigg, 1992: 4). Specific improvements to working conditions, social protection systems and provision for the needs of employees as carers may be introduced through the European Union's social policies if not by national governments. It will, however, be much more difficult to address entrenched assumptions about the gendered divisions of caring work within and outside the home, by paid and unpaid carers. Such unresolved issues ensure that community care will remain firmly on the agenda of *women and social policy* into the twenty-first century.

10 Men's violence and relationship breakdown: can violence be dealt with as an exception to the rule?

Carol-Ann Hooper

This chapter concerns the implications of recent policies which redefine the framework for regulating relations between ex-partners and their children after relationship breakdown, for women leaving men violent to themselves and/or their children. The Children Act 1989, the Child Support Act 1991 and the proposals for reform of the divorce law are examined. In these policies the problem of men's violence to women and children in families has been dealt with (if at all) as an exceptional circumstance. While the Children Act 1989 places violence against children at the centre of its concerns (in its public law, if less in its private law, provisions), violence against women (which has implications too for children) is not addressed. The Child Support Act 1991 recognised the problem of violence (after lobbying from women's groups) only as an exceptional circumstance, which may entitle women on means-tested benefits to exemption from the requirement to co-operate with the pursuit of their ex-partners for maintenance payments where there is a risk of 'harm or undue distress' to them or their children. The proposals for reform of the divorce law argue that the need for protection from violence is a separate matter from the legal process leading to divorce itself.

Feminist research has, however, highlighted the limitations of treating men's violence to women and children as exceptional, a deviation from the norm, and drawn attention to the extent to which it is, rather, embedded within the norms of contemporary patriarchal social relations. Feminist activists and researchers have also drawn attention to the ways in which state responses frequently fail to provide appropriate help to women leaving violent men, in the areas of housing provision (Bull, 1991),

146

social work (Maynard, 1985) and the criminal and civil law (see Dobash and Dobash, 1992), and the resulting lack of confidence women have in the state in this context. An approach to the problem of men's violence against women and children which treats it as an exceptional circumstance is problematic, for two reasons. First, the state's role in defining what counts as an exception gives it a gatekeeping role in relation to women's claims of violence, which may result in excluding some women from necessary protection. Second, the implications of the main policy provisions for the problem of men's violence against women and children can too easily remain unaddressed if provision for cases of violence is added on as an afterthought. The result is in effect a tokenistic response, which appears to offer protection to women and children from men's violence but at the same time may allow the conditions which foster violence to continue unchecked, or indeed to worsen.

The chapter first makes the case for attention to the problem of men's violence to women and children in families and reviews briefly what is known about it: its nature and extent, how it (and women's responses to it) can be understood and how state agencies have responded. It then outlines the ways in which the framework of family law has changed over recent years and considers the evidence so far available on the implications of these changes for women leaving violent men. Finally, some suggestions are offered for developing a policy framework which might be more genuinely protective and preventative.

The problem of men's violence to women and children

Iris Young (1990) has argued that violence is one of the five faces of oppression, along with exploitation, marginalisation, powerlessness and cultural imperialism. In a number of contexts, violence is directed against women and other oppressed groups, ethnic minorities, gay men and lesbians, for example, as a systematic social practice; in other words, it is directed at individuals because of their membership of these social groups. For women, the home is one of these contexts. What makes men's violence to women and children in the home a 'face of oppression' rather than an individual act of bad behaviour is that the social context makes the use of violence in that relationship possible and acceptable. In focusing on men's violence to women and children in families, I am not assuming that women are a homogeneous group nor that women are not sometimes violent themselves. Women's experiences differ in numerous ways. Nevertheless, it is useful to focus on a core dimension of oppression, accepting that individuals experience it in different measure and that their position in relation to all social divisions (in particular class, age, race, religion, ability, sexual orientation as well as gender) influences that experience profoundly. In addition while women are sometimes violent to men, to other women and (more often) to children in families, men's violence to women and children in families is a distinctive problem because of the influence of the other 'faces of oppression' on its context. Women's marginalisation in the labour market, their exploitation as unpaid carers of children and others, their relative powerlessness in the public worlds of policy and law and the patriarchal norms against which their behaviour is often judged in those public worlds all result in a quite different context of options for women leaving violent men from those which face men leaving violent women. That context differs too for different women, influenced again by their position in relation to other divisions. However, in the context of the break-down of heterosexual relationships (the main focus of the policies considered in this chapter)[1] gender divisions come very much to the centre of the stage.

Defining what constitutes violence is not unproblematic – either within families or in the wider world of public policy and research. Definitions are socially constructed and therefore variable, involving judgements which are affected by community and cultural norms and by personal and professional values and expectations. As Liz Kelly (1988) has argued, definitions are contested within the context of male dominance, where it is in men's interests as a group and as the main perpetrators of violence for such defini-tions to be as limited as possible. Hence feminist activism and research have sought to problematise dominant definitions and to establish broader, more inclusive definitions which more accurately represent women's reality, identifying the wide range of be-haviours – physical, verbal, sexual, emotional and psychological – which women experi-ence as violence. Hence too, however, women themselves often minimise their own experiences, partly as a way of managing the tensions between dominant definitions and their own experiential reality, and partly in response to their anticipation of not being taken seriously by others (Kelly and Radford, 1990/1). Similar processes can also result in women minimising their children's experiences of abuse, although where sexual abuse is concerned additional difficulties of obtaining and interpreting evidence may also inhibit the recognition of abuse (Hooper, 1992).

There is no nationally representative study to indicate the extent of men's violence in the home. One recent survey based on a random sample of households in Islington, however, found that over a third of women reported having experienced some form of violence from a partner at some point in their lives (Mooney, 1993). Further evidence indicates that in the context of relationship breakdown violence is not a rare circum-stance. Bradshaw and Millar's (1991) nationally representative survey of lone parents found that 20 per cent gave violence as one of the reasons for separating from their most recent partner (13 per cent gave it as the main reason, 7 per cent as a supple-mentary reason), and the researchers suggest that the survey may well have underesti-mated the extent of violence in these relationships. Studies of court records suggest that the majority of petitions for divorce filed by women on the grounds of 'unreason-able behaviour' involve violence (although some women who have experienced vio-lence also seek divorce on other grounds) (Borkowski *et al.*, 1983; Law Commission, 1990). In 1991, 40 per cent of all divorces involved women as petitioners using the behaviour ground (OPCS, 1991). Extrapolating from the various sources, it is likely that at least a third of all divorces involve women seeking divorce in response partly to violence against themselves or their children.

How can men's violence to women and children in families be explained? This is a complex question, given the different forms violence can take and the interaction between individual (conscious and unconscious) and social dimensions at play in any specific incident. As Gordon (1989) has argued, violence in families is always both a personal interaction and an expression of social and cultural stresses and tensions, reflecting inequalities of sex, generation, class and race. Here only the social dimensions are considered, focusing on three which have been highlighted and/or debated by feminists and/or which are particularly pertinent to the policies which are the focus of this chapter: gender relations, poverty and family structure.

The central contribution of feminist thinking on men's violence to women in families has been to highlight the ways in which gender inequalities in society make it possible by constraining women's access to resources and options for independence from men, and male-dominated institutions make it acceptable by implicitly or explicitly condoning it, failing to intervene effectively to protect women from men's violence in the name of preserving 'family privacy', and perpetuating a construction of male authority and female dependence within families which allows men a sense of entitlement to behave in proprietary fashion towards 'their' women. The common justification given by men who murder their wives (or ex-wives) for their behaviour – 'if I can't have you, no one can' – exemplifies this attitude to women, as men's property to be kept under control, *in extremis* (Wilson and Daly, 1992). The same sense of entitlement underlies lesser incidents of domestic violence, however. These occur in the context of conflicts over men's expectations of women's domestic work and availability and over men's sexual jealousy and possessiveness in particular, conflicts in which women's struggles for autonomy (or 'insubordination') are met with men's use of violence to maintain or reassert their own power, control and authority (Dobash and Dobash, 1992).

While gender inequalities in the labour market and consequently in access to social security benefits and housing (documented elsewhere in this book) clearly affect women's options for leaving, recent feminist analyses have focused also on the role played by the construction of gender difference both in relation to men's propensity to be violent and to women's reluctance to leave. Goldner *et al.* (1990) have argued that in relationships in which men abuse women, gender stereotypes are adhered to in rigid and exaggerated form. Battering, they suggest, may be 'a man's attempt to reassert gender difference and gender dominance, when his terror of not being different enough from "his" woman threaten to overtake him' (p. 348), in a context in which to blur the boundaries of gender difference is to risk the humiliation of losing patriarchal power and privilege, and in which aggression restores a sense of masculine identity. Similarly (or rather differently), women's commitment to staying, and lack of commitment to their own safety in doing so, may reflect a sense of self in which the ability to sustain relationships is central, which in turn reflects the centrality of caring to the construction of femininity in contemporary society, and its damaging consequences for women when care is extended to others but not to self. Evidence that many women who return to violent men cite as important reasons a continued sense of responsibility for them, a desire to give them another chance and the belief that children need both parents supports this analysis (Binney *et al.*, 1981).

Men's violence to women and children occurs across class and race and evidence as to whether these divisions influence its prevalence (or simply its reporting and labelling) is mixed and inconclusive. Arguments that economic deprivation contributes to violence which fail also to take into account gender relations are clearly inadequate since women are more vulnerable to poverty yet men are more often violent. Lack of resources, however, may increase the potential for conflicts between men and women in the home – over money, children and space, for example – conflicts which are responded to in gendered ways. In addition, male unemployment and the loss of the breadwinner role, and experiences of powerlessness or victimisation at work or elsewhere, may threaten masculine identity in ways for which men seek compensation through aggressive control of women. Perhaps most clearly, however, women's economic dependence on men within families and poverty as lone parents affects their ability to protect themselves and their children from violent men – partners, ex-partners and new partners (Strube, 1988; Mooney, 1993; Mooney and Young, 1993).

The New Right has made much of data which it is claimed demonstrate that children are at higher risk of abuse in non-traditional families (especially stepfather families, married or cohabiting), using this to reconstitute the problem of child abuse as attributable to the breakdown of the traditional family (Gledhill *et al.*, 1989; Willetts, 1993; Whelan, 1994) rather than, as feminists have argued, to the power relations of traditional families (Herman and Hirschman, 1981; Stark and Flitcraft, 1988; Gordon, 1989). This argument has been based largely on reported cases and for the most part on cases placed on child protection registers – data which should be treated with great caution. Records frequently misrepresent the family situation of the child at the time of abuse, for example recording the child as living in a lone-parent family when the abuse was perpetrated by the natural father before the parents separated (Andrews, 1994). Furthermore, statistics on registered cases may well reflect greater willingness amongst professionals to suspect stepfathers or mothers' boyfriends of abuse and the lesser conflicts of loyalty children (and their mothers) may feel about disclosing such abuse than abuse by natural fathers.

There is some evidence from other sources that living with a stepfather is associated with increased risk of child sexual abuse, both by step- or substitute fathers, and by other men (Russell, 1984; Andrews, 1994). The significance of this connection should not be overstated, however. There is much clearer evidence of a correlation between domestic violence and physical child abuse (Bowker *et al.*, 1988; Stark and Flitcraft, 1988); the negative impacts of witnessing domestic violence on children suggest that domestic violence itself constitutes a form of emotional abuse of children (Jaffe *et al.*, 1990), and numerically more girls are sexually abused by natural fathers than by step- or substitute fathers (Russell, 1984). Arguing for divorce to be made more difficult in order to protect children from potential stepfathers is misguided, at best. If such an outcome were achieved it would be likely to place far more children at risk than it protected.

The extent to which stepfather families do create increased risks for children is unclear. Assuming they do (to some extent), a number of processes may be involved. Some evidence suggests that men who have been involved in childcare and nurturing during the early years of a child's life are less likely to abuse them (Parker and Parker,

1986). While this applies to both natural and substitute fathers, the latter are less likely to have been involved in the early care of stepchildren. In addition, the stepfather–stepchild relationship may be a difficult one for a number of reasons: its cultural devaluation in the context of the idealisation of the 'natural family' and the emphasis placed on mothers as central for their children's welfare, the expectation of establishing an instant parent–child relationship without the history of continuous intimacy through which parent–child relationships usually develop, the emotional complexity of family transitions and the tenuousness in law of such relationships. The ambiguity – even irrelevancy – of the role may be seriously at odds with men's expectation of authority in the home, leading some to attempt to assert their authority with violence (Dimnik, 1987).

Women do not easily go public with complaints of their own or their children's victimisation from their partners. When seeking help, they often do so tentatively and ambivalently, inhibited by feelings of shame, guilt and self-blame at the 'failure' of their relationship or their ability to protect their children, by a reluctance to breach their own values of family privacy, loyalty and obligation, by fears of repercussions from the violent man and/or other family members, and by scepticism about the likely helpfulness of the agencies they approach. While these fears occur across class and race, ethnic minority women may have additional fears – of breaching community as well as family loyalties and of encountering racist responses (Mama, 1989) – and both ethnic minority and working-class women may fear discriminatory and pathologising judgements of their parenting.

Fears about the responses of agencies are well founded. While some women clearly do get the help they need (usually after a number of attempts), responses from police, courts, housing departments and social security offices are variable and frequently inadequate (see Dobash and Dobash, 1992; Morley, 1993, for reviews of relevant research). Women's accounts of violence are frequently not believed or taken seriously, their own behaviour is often pathologised, and loopholes are often found by which to exclude or defer their claims (e.g. for rehousing). These problems reflect the role the welfare state plays in mediating gender, 'race' and class divisions within a patriarchal and racially structured capitalist society (Williams, 1989) (as one site – or rather, a multiplicity of sites – on which struggles must be fought in male-dominated institutions for women's, and especially ethnic minority women's, voices to be heard and needs to be met), the influence of economic constraints and the consequent pressures on agency workers to delimit need, and reluctance to intervene in the 'private' sphere of the family. While the value accorded to family privacy often leads to insufficient attention to women's needs for help, at the same time women report feeling degraded and humiliated by the intrusion into privacy which contact with the Department of Social Security often involves, with its efforts to reinforce women's dependency on men rather than the state (Dean and Taylor-Gooby, 1992; Kirkwood, 1993).

The common experience of responses which do not meet women's needs for protection from violent men (from formal and informal networks) has a number of consequences. First, the institutional frustration of their efforts to leave (especially difficulties in finding affordable accommodation) is one of the main reasons women stay with or return to violent men (Binney *et al.*, 1981). Second, while some women persist until they find the help they need, others' expectations of help decline to the point where they become reluctant to ask (Hoff, 1990). Third, the ineffectiveness of state responses means women develop their own personal strategies for protection, in particular attempting to keep their whereabouts unknown to their ex-partners (Kirkwood, 1993). Such strategies are adopted because separation does not necessarily stop violence. Nevertheless separation certainly helps, and the effects of policy both on the negotiation of decisions to separate or divorce and on arrangements post-separation are important in influencing women's ability to escape violent men. The changing framework of family law which regulates relations on separation and/or divorce is considered next.

The changing framework of family law

The Children Act 1989 in its private law provisions redefined the framework for parents' ongoing relationships with their children after separation or divorce. The old terms 'custody' and 'access' were abolished and replaced by the concept of 'parental responsibility' which is retained by both parents after divorce, and four new orders (under Section 8 – residence, contact, prohibited steps and specific issue orders) which can be made by courts if parents are unable to reach their own agreements about which parent the children will live with, how often they will see the other parent and so on. The Child Support Act 1991 set out a new framework for the assessment and collection of maintenance from non-resident parents (or absent parents as they are called in this context), based on the use of a standard formula by the newly established Child Support Agency, to replace the previous system of discretionary awards made by the courts. The proposals for reform of the divorce law – which it is not yet certain will be implemented – would replace the existing five grounds for divorce[2] by a single ground of 'irretrievable breakdown', to be proved by requiring couples to wait a year – a 'cooling-off period' – before being granted a divorce, and urging them to use mediation services during this period to resolve conflicts where possible, or at least to reach agreement on post-divorce arrangements.

There has been a mixture of motivations behind these policy changes, including economic restructuring (to reduce the costs of social security to lone parents on benefit and of legal aid to divorcing couples), humanitarian concerns (to reduce the distress children and adults may experience at divorce) and patriarchal restructuring (in the traditional sense of reinforcing the role of fatherhood as well as women's economic dependence on men). Despite increasing emphasis in Conservative rhetoric on strengthening the traditional family and deterring family breakdown, policies have not (as yet) reflected a straightforward attempt to turn back the tide of family and social change by making divorce more difficult (although the divorce proposals do make the prevention of divorce where possible an explicit aim). The Children Act 1989 and the Child Support Act 1991 have attempted to influence behaviour after separation and divorce (to maintain parental responsibilities despite it) rather than to influence the incidence of divorce itself.

The two Acts are not a wholly consistent package, differing in their concepts of parental responsibility, the role accorded to the state and their approach to children's welfare (Clarke *et al.*, 1993). Equally important, the government have argued that the two areas of responsibility they cover are unrelated, that is, that enforcing the obligation to pay maintenance has no implications for arrangements regarding contact, a view which research suggests does not accord with parental practice.[3]

Two consistent themes which are particularly significant in considering the implications of these changes for women are the increased emphasis on parental responsibility and the reduced role of the courts. While parental responsibility has different meanings in different contexts, in both the Children Act and the Child Support Act it is lifelong and irrevocable (except by giving the child up for adoption) and regardless of the marital status of the biological parents (although unmarried fathers do not automatically have it under the Children Act as they do under the Child Support Act). The concept has been promoted as an unquestionable good (who could be in favour of parental irresponsibility?). However, in contemporary New Right discourse it is linked to an individualist philosophy in which having children is seen as a personal choice and hence an individual (parental) rather than a social responsibility, and to the government's aim of reducing the role of the state (and increasing the role of the family) in the provision of welfare. It is also a concept which is gendered in its impact, since both during and after marriage women still bear the primary responsibility for the day-to-day care of children, and hence the majority of resident parents (or parents with care) continue to be women, and the majority of non-resident (or absent) parents continue to be men.

An emphasis on parental responsibility is often linked to a declared commitment to child welfare, as if the former (whatever its meaning) necessarily achieves the latter (which is, of course, equally variable in meaning). In the context of the Child Support Act this commitment is clearly empty, since the majority of children whose mothers are on benefits receive none of the maintenance their fathers pay (which is deducted pound for pound from income support), and the fathers of children whose mothers are not on benefits are not required to pay (since co-operation is only compulsory for women on income support, family credit or disability working allowance). In the context of the Children Act, children's welfare is to be treated as paramount. However, its private law provisions were strongly influenced by a particular construction of children's welfare which equates children's needs in the context of parental divorce with ongoing relationships with both parents. The belief that contact with non-resident fathers is necessarily beneficial to children pervades court and mediation practice, despite the evidence that the two most important factors in mediating the impact of divorce on children are lone mothers' well-being and the protection of children from exposure to conflict, and that the impact of contact with non-resident fathers can be positive, negative or neither (Furstenburg and Cherlin, 1991; see also Hooper, 1994, for further discussion). Smart (1989) has argued that this redefinition of children's needs in the context of parental divorce reflects the overlapping influence of the fathers' rights movement and the New Right – as such, it is closely interwoven with patriarchal restructuring.

Both Acts also aim to reduce the role of the courts in relationship breakdown (as do the divorce proposals). In the Children Act 1989 this represents a reduction in state regulation of family relationships and an increased trend towards their private ordering, since parents are expected to reach agreements between them if possible. Both court-based and independent mediation services are expanding rapidly to help them do so, and the courts can make an order only if it is judged better for the child than making no order. However, decisions covered by the Child Support Act have been taken over by the bureaucratic decision-making machinery of the Child Support Agency, and explicitly increase state regulation of family relationships (albeit with the aim of reducing state expenditure). The divorce reforms too would increase state regulation if all divorcing couples were to be required to receive professional advice. The reduced role of the courts is not therefore a simple rolling back of the state as much as a change in the form of state regulation.

While formal justice does not always serve women well, it does have some advantages over the informal justice of mediation. In legal disputes, each party has separate representation, a solicitor to represent their interests and to negotiate on their behalf, someone 'on their side'. Because of their partisan role solicitors have tended to be found the most helpful of all agencies contacted by women leaving violent men (Binney *et al.*, 1981). In mediation, this is (usually) replaced by a single mediator, operating in relation to the couple together, from a stance of professional 'neutrality'. This stance of neutrality conceals the values and beliefs which are purveyed through mediation (Bottomley, 1985). Piper (1993) has argued that mediation is underpinned by a particular construction of parental responsibility, in which pre-separation responsibilities are accorded little significance, and in which agreement between parents post-separation is seen as a desirable outcome *per se*, and indicative of joint responsibility for children (whatever the arrangements agreed). This construction systematically disadvantages women because of their greater responsibilities for the care of children (pre- and post-separation). Women's responsibilities for children and the role of caring in feminine identity also make women more susceptible to images presented as in children's interests, leading some to 'give in' to agreements which later seem unjust. Hence informal justice tends to reinforce existing inequalities, although there is considerable variability in both practice and outcome (Piper, 1993).

These developments raise concerns about women's ability to leave violent men which are considered in more detail below. While different provision has been made for such women in the Child Support Act and could be extended in other areas, for example through exemption from mediation (Hester and Pearson, 1993), the fact that women do not easily define their own or their children's experience as violence or tell others of them, and that they are not always believed when they do, means that they are also affected by approaches to divorcing couples in general.

The Children Act 1989

For women leaving violent men, arrangements regarding the children's contact with their fathers have implications for the children's safety (obviously) and also for their own. Violence does not necessarily stop at separation and violent men may use contact with their children to exercise control over their ex-partners. Hester and Radford (1992), in a study of women's experiences of access arrangements after domestic violence (pre-Children Act), found a number of tactics were reported, including abuse of their mother at 'hand-over' time, abduction of the children and their use as hostages, grilling children for information about their mothers and challenging existing arrangements in order to harass women via the courts.

In addition, a history and/or ongoing threat of violence may affect both the process and the outcome of negotiations – meetings for mediation/conciliation may result in incidents of violence during the meeting and/or after, and the power and control dynamics of the relationship may make genuinely negotiated agreements difficult (Hester and Pearson, 1993). The role of mediation in circumstances of domestic violence has been much debated in the United States, with some arguing it is wholly inappropriate and others arguing it can have positive outcomes in some cases but only if mediators are specially trained to identify and handle domestic violence cases.[4] So far there has been little attention to the issue in the United Kingdom, and Hester and Pearson (1993) report a common lack of knowledge about the dynamics and implications of domestic violence amongst mediators, resulting in variable and inconsistent practice. While some individuals have developed practical ways of ensuring safety for women and children, both during the process (e.g. seeing partners separately) and in the aftermath (e.g. recommending neutral territory for hand-overs so women can keep their addresses secret and/or supervised access), there is no consistent policy either on identifying or on handling cases of domestic violence as yet, and a tendency to minimise both its extent and effects (Hester and Pearson, 1993; WAFE, 1993).

While the principle of prioritising children's welfare gives the courts the power to prevent contact with a non-resident parent (or to specify the conditions in which it may take place) if it is thought to be harmful to the child, circumstances justifying the stopping of contact are regarded as exceptional. This was so prior to the Children Act 1989, but has become more so. Research suggests that women commonly share the widespread belief that children's contact with their fathers is important and attempt to maintain it where possible, despite the difficulties it can often create for themselves and some reservations about its impact on children (Hester and Radford, 1992; Clarke *et al.*, 1993). Where they attempt to stop or restrict contact in response to men's violence, however, and fathers in return apply for a contact order through the courts, women face considerable obstacles. These include the tendency of the courts to minimise the extent and effects of men's violence (e.g. by disregarding the effects on children of violence to their mothers) and to pathologise women (e.g. by attributing their concerns about their children's safety to their own histories of abuse and/or hostility to ex-partners), the difficulty of gathering evidence to substantiate women's concerns (especially where the sexual abuse of a child is suspected), the presumption in favour of maintaining children's contact with fathers, which can result in a 'naive optimism' about the ability of fathers to learn childcare skills post-divorce through contact even if they had none previously (Hester and Radford, 1992), insufficient resources (e.g. access centres) to provide safe supervised contact, and a failure to take women's own safety seriously (e.g. revealing their addresses to ex-partners as part of the contact order). As a result Women's Aid Federation England (WAFE) (1993) reports that contact orders are placing women and children at risk from violent men.

The Child Support Act 1991

While the Child Support Act has been described as having a 'convulsive effect on relationships between parents, between new partners and both directly and indirectly on children' (NACAB, 1994: 96), the impact of the imposition of a bureaucratically regulated system of financial redistribution on the complex area of family relationships is difficult to assess in detail after only a year of implementation. There is much that is not yet known. Nevertheless, the Child Support Agency's own report on its first year and the reports of voluntary organisations monitoring its impact suggest some concerns in relation both to the provision for exemption from the requirement to co-operate (without the imposition of a benefit penalty) for women who fear violence from their ex-partners, and in relation to the wider implications for violence of the reforms themselves.

In the first year of its operation, the Child Support Agency (CSA) considered 65,000 cases in relation to exemption from the requirement to co-operate (of a total of 858,000 returned Maintenance Application Forms (MAFs)). In 32,000 of these, the case for exemption was accepted, in about 700 the penalty was applied and in 14,200 the parents with care eventually co-operated (the remainder were still undecided when these figures were produced) (CSA, 1994). Exemption has therefore been granted in under 4 per cent of all cases, many of these for reasons other than 'harm or undue distress' (CPAG, 1994).[5] This is lower than might be expected given the prevalence of violence against women and children. Several factors may have deflated the numbers. First, cases pursued by the Agency have tended to involve men who were easily traceable and these may be disproportionately those involved in more amicable separations (NACAB, 1994). Second, the 14,200 parents who co-operated after initially applying for exemption may include many who do face risks but agreed to co-operate as a result of pressure from Agency staff unwilling to accept their case and/or reluctance to face further intrusive questioning. While some staff are reported to have handled cases involving violence sensitively, voluntary organisations also report cases in which women have been asked for documentary proof (despite the guidance that the woman's word should be accepted 'unless . . . inherently implausible') and in which women's concerns have been excluded by the imposition of a narrow and inflexible interpretation of 'harm and undue distress' (excluding psychological abuse, for example) (NACAB, 1994; NCOPF, 1994). The guidance issued to Child Support Officers leaves room for discretion and hence practice varies both between different areas and within any one area (CPAG, 1994). Third, other women may not have applied for exemption, as a result either of lack of knowledge of its existence or of distrust in the Agency to take their concerns seriously and offer the protection they need. Clarke *et al.* (1993) note that lone mothers sometimes conflated the naming of the father and the authorising of maintenance, believing (inaccurately) that if the DSS already knew the father's name there was nothing the woman could do to stop action being taken to pursue him for maintenance. Voluntary organisations have noted that many lone mothers remain uninformed about their rights to exemption, despite widespread awareness of the threat of the benefit penalty (NACAB, 1994; NCOPF, 1994). Some women appear to have withdrawn their benefit claims altogether rather than risk the Agency pursuing their ex-partners for maintenance (CPAG, 1994; NACAB, 1994).[6]

The evidence so far suggests that in the context of the present system, the exemption clause as currently implemented provides inadequate protection for women attempting to escape violent men. In addition, the CSA may itself exacerbate the problems of men's violence in a number of ways. Qualitative studies suggest that men frequently expect the payment of maintenance to buy them some *quid pro quo* rights, whether this is in relation to the mother (to exercise some control over how the money is spent, for example) or in relation to the children (to contact and/or other forms of participation in their lives) (Clarke *et al.*, 1993; Burgoyne and Millar, 1994; Skinner, 1994). Enforcing the CSA's system of maintenance therefore has implications for relations between men, women and children, and may in effect extend the web of 'private patriarchy' (Walby, 1990a) beyond relationship breakdown.

In Clark *et al.*'s (1993) study, lone mothers anticipated that maintenance assessments would result in verbal abuse and/or physical violence to them from their ex-partners, and some men have indeed responded with violence in this way (CPAG, 1994). The Agency claims to provide a buffer by acting as go-between between ex-partners, but can offer no protection to women from their ex-partners' hostility if the men know or can trace the women's whereabouts. Violence from men towards ex-partners in this context is not simply a response to a demand for money (in the manner of responding to increased gas bills, where the gas company might be thought to be the appropriate target); rather, it is likely to be both a response to the threatened undermining of men's ability to perform the breadwinning role in second families and an expression of a sense of entitlement and proprietariness towards ex-partners and their children, reinforced by the extension of the breadwinning role for them beyond relationship breakdown.

In addition, the maintenance formula's inclusion of a carer allowance (to recognise the indirect costs of caring) explicitly reinforces women's economic dependency on men (and its link with caring responsibilities), again extending it beyond relationship breakdown. Clarke *et al.* (1993) report strong opposition to this aspect in particular amongst the lone mothers they interviewed (pre-implementation of the Child Support Act) for that reason, alongside considerable ambivalence about the receipt of maintenance for children which was perceived both as men's necessary obligation and as impeding women's ability to escape men's control (Clarke *et al.*, 1993). Women's economic dependency on men is also increased in cases where women have refused to co-operate with the Agency after reaching private agreements with their ex-partners to make up the income lost by the imposition of the benefit penalty. Women who have withdrawn from benefit altogether in order to avoid their ex-partners being pursued for maintenance will thereby be more vulnerable to economic dependence on new partners (CPAG, 1994).

While some have argued that children may benefit if reinforcing fathers' financial obligations after divorce also encourages them to stay involved in their children's lives, the effects on father–child relationships appear to be more complex and variable. Some fathers have been unable to continue existing arrangements for contact because the costs of contact visits have not so far been recognised in the maintenance formula, and some contact visits have been made more difficult by the tensions in second families created by maintenance assessments (Clarke *et al.*, 1994). Other fathers have wanted to resume contact after long absences from their children's lives, in exchange for maintenance payments. Others still have threatened to apply for residence orders or persuaded children to move in with them (or stay more with them than with the other parent) in order to avoid maintenance payments by becoming the parent with care (CPAG, 1994; NACAB, 1994; NCOPF, 1994). Increased contact with children motivated by a desire to reduce maintenance liability or as a *quid pro quo* with reluctant ex-partners is unlikely to be in children's interests; rather, it may increase children's exposure to parental conflict and their vulnerability to poor quality care if not abuse.

In the future, it is possible also that anticipation of their maintenance obligations may make some men reluctant to leave the household when women wish to separate or divorce. As Millar suggests in Chapter 4, research on the distribution of resources within households has shown that the assumption embedded in the 'family wage' ideology, namely that resources are shared equitably, is not necessarily valid (e.g. Pahl, 1989). Yet the CSA attempts to impose just this sharing between households, and is able to regulate and enforce breadwinner obligations in a way which is impossible within households. Some men may therefore prefer to keep their dependants within the same household to maintain their own control over financial resources (as has happened with some children post-separation). The carer allowance in particular may increase men's resistance to leaving and/or their hostility to ex-partners when they do, since Burgoyne and Millar (1994) reported strong opposition from separated fathers to paying maintenance for ex-partners (as opposed to for children), especially where it was the woman who had wanted the separation. The rigidity of the maintenance formula, which allows no adjustments to take into account previous property settlements, will also reduce women's claims on the matrimonial home if they separate[7] – at the same time as their claim to priority for permanent rehousing is lost in changes to provision for homeless families. The Child Support Act may thus significantly increase the difficulties for women and children attempting to leave violent men.

In addition, the explicit priority given biological children by the Act may have consequences for stepfather–stepchild relationships. Stepchildren are expected to be financially supported primarily by their biological fathers, potentially increasing the ambiguity and devaluation of the stepfather role. Some stepfathers' capacity to support stepchildren has also been depleted by the enforcement of their financial obligations to biological children. If stepfathers' sense of their ability to perform a breadwinner role in their current families and of responsibility towards stepchildren is further undermined, the latter's vulnerability to abuse may be increased.

Further research is needed to establish the way in which the Child Support Act is affecting relationships and decision making within families; however, these aspects are crucial in considering the implications of the Act for women, and merit further attention. The distributive paradigm which predominates in social policy – with its focus on who gains and who loses in financial terms – is insufficient to capture the impacts on relations between men and women, parents and children which may significantly affect the vulnerability of women and children to violence and their ability to escape it. Women in employment may gain financially from the receipt of maintenance (depending on the level of their ex-partners' income) but yet may lose in terms of the ability to control their own lives or the impact on their children. Such a gain is therefore not necessarily equivalent to a gain in income from other sources, the labour market or the state.

The distributive impacts also, however, have implications for violence. While the Child Support Act has been welcomed by some for redistributing income from men to women (NCOPF, 1994), the reality is somewhat more complex. The majority (70 per cent) of lone mothers are dependent on income support and hence currently receive no benefit from their ex-partners' maintenance payments. Indeed, some lone mothers have been made worse off through the imposition of the benefit penalty, the loss of passported benefits for those lifted off income support (e.g. free prescriptions and school meals), the loss of informal payments from ex-partners and/or withdrawal from benefit altogether. For these women, their difficulties in escaping violent ex-partners may be increased by their lack of resources. In addition, since repartnering and employment offer the two main routes out of poverty, increased poverty may make lone mothers more vulnerable to repartnering with abusive men and/or taking employment without providing good-quality substitute care for children, influencing both their own and their children's vulnerability to violence.

While some changes have been made to benefits for those in work in order to make re-entry into the labour market more attractive for lone mothers by increasing incentives, the heavy reliance on means-testing to achieve this policy aim creates problems of complexity and insecurity (Millar, 1996). In the absence of broader policies to increase the availability of good-quality, affordable childcare, improve training and education for women returners and create secure job opportunities at reasonable rates of pay, such changes are likely to make little impact on lone mothers' poverty. In reality the redistribution of income is occurring primarily from low-income families to the state – the result, the increased stresses of poverty amongst low income households (stepfamily as well as lone-mother households).

The divorce proposals

The proposals for reform to the divorce law have received a mixed response within the Conservative party. Despite one of the stated objectives being to save 'saveable marriages' (Lord Chancellor's Department, 1993: 3), the removal of fault from the grounds for divorce has been seen by some as inconsistent with the government's (already shaky) claim to the moral high ground on family values. At the time of writing, it is not clear what changes (if any) will become law. However, in their current form, the proposals raise a number of concerns in relation to women's ability to leave violent men.

The Green Paper argues that it is the civil law remedies which give protection against violence and harassment by former spouses, rather than divorce itself. These remedies do not at present offer very much protection, however. Barron's (1990) recent study found that only about half the women who applied for civil protection through the courts achieved what they asked for, and of those who did achieve an order or 'undertaking', again only about half found it effective in preventing further violence or harassment from their partners. Recommendations from the Law Commission for reform of the civil law on injunctions may improve the situation somewhat but are unlikely to guarantee protection so long as judicial discretion remains (Morley, 1993).

It is unlikely that the divorce process itself is irrelevant to women's ability to escape violent men. The fault grounds – which allow divorce quickly, with the average time from submission of petition to granting of decree absolute being six months – are used far more by women than men, more by lower socio-economic groups than higher, and more by couples with children than by couples without (Law Commission, 1990). Those with fewer resources appear much less likely to use the separation grounds, probably because they are less able to afford separate accommodation during the waiting period. The requirement that all couples wait a year would place women who cannot find affordable alternative accommodation during this period at increased risk, especially in the light of evidence that women's declared intentions of leaving often prompt further violence from violent men in their attempts to re-establish control (Wilson and Daly, 1992). Given that the purpose of the year's wait is to hold open the possibility of reconciliation, local authorities may become more reluctant to rehouse women in the interim. For women who can separate during the waiting period, their personal strategies of protection may be made more difficult by the wait for the divorce itself.

The proposals stop short (just) of making mediation/conciliation compulsory. They suggest, however, a compulsory first interview for all those considering divorce, in which information would be given about divorce and its consequences, the law, marriage guidance and mediation, and in which couples thought to have saveable marriages would be recommended to use marriage guidance and others would be encouraged to use mediation to reach agreement on ancillary matters rather than to litigate. The year's wait is then intended to encourage reflection, on the assumption that couples currently abandon their marriages too lightly, without considering the consequences for either themselves or their children. Where women leaving violent men are concerned, the evidence suggests rather the opposite. Binney *et al.* (1981) found that the average length of time women had suffered violence from their partners before leaving was seven years. The emphasis placed in the proposed changes on encouraging couples to accept joint responsibility for the marriage breakdown and to focus on their children's needs rather than their own may exacerbate just the self-blame and self-denial which make it difficult already for women to leave violent men. This risk could be reduced if the potential dangers of mediation in the context of domestic violence, raised earlier, were recognised. However, the current proposals express concern that claims of domestic violence may be 'exploited' to avoid considering the merits of mediation which does not suggest a climate receptive to prioritising women's safety. While women who can afford to pay the legal costs of divorce themselves may be able to avoid mediation if they wish, those who need legal aid may not. It is proposed that legal aid be available on a means-tested basis, with the proviso that it can be withdrawn from those deemed to be 'behaving unreasonably'. 'Unreasonable behaviour' is clearly subject to interpretation, which may be influenced by gendered expectations of behaviour. In addition, women may feel pressurised to participate in mediation against their better judgement for fear that refusal to do so will result in the loss of legal aid.

Conclusions

The analysis in this chapter suggests that there are dangers in relying on exceptions to the rule to protect women and children from violent men. Neither the Child Support Agency's implementation of its exemption clause nor the courts' decisions on contact orders and injunctions appear to offer effective protection. Such provision could undoubtedly be made more effective, with a proactive approach involving public education, screening to identify cases of violence and education and training for the gatekeepers. Exceptions could also be extended to other areas, exempting women from mediation in circumstances involving violence, for example. Even effective exceptions, however, might not remove altogether the impact of the rules themselves on women leaving violent men. Women may acquire information about these policies not tailored to their specific circumstances, which may affect their sense of options for independence from male partners. Their sense of what alternatives to their current situation are possible may in turn affect their ability to define that situation as unacceptable.

Furthermore, to focus on exceptions diverts attention from the nature of the rules themselves and their potential for exacerbating the problem of men's violence. An alternative way forward therefore is to consider the framing of policy so as to enable women to protect themselves and their children from violence as a priority, not as an afterthought. In the Child Support Act, exemption is only necessary because co-operation was made compulsory for women receiving means-tested benefits. Yet the principle that fathers should continue to support their children financially after divorce has widespread support – 90 per cent of men and 95 per cent of women agreed with it in the British Social Attitudes survey of 1992. A system perceived to be fair and effective would be likely to attract a high level of voluntary co-operation from lone mothers.[8] A voluntary system would extend the choices already available to women not on benefits to all, and would place the decision as to whether to pursue maintenance or not in the hands of the person most able to judge the effects on family relationships, the parent with care. Similarly the implicit compulsion to use mediation in the divorce proposals creates both a two-tier approach (since women who can afford solicitors' fees will still be able to use them) and an urgent need for exemption for women leaving violent men. Yet it is widely recognised that mediation is only likely to be effective if it is voluntary.

Exceptions are also made necessary by the aim of preserving either a particular family form, the married, two-biological-parent family as preferable (as in the divorce proposals) or as much of its responsibilities as possible despite its changing form (as in the Children Act and Child Support Act). The flag of children's needs is frequently waved to justify such an aim, yet the impact on children of divorce, of lone parenthood and of ongoing relationships with fathers after divorce is highly variable. The negative impacts of divorce (where found) are attributable to a large extent to parental conflict (pre- as well as post-separation) and poverty, and children appear to adjust best when their resident parent is able to take control of her own life and decisions.[9] Requiring women who have decided on divorce to wait for a year, compelling them (explicitly or implicitly) to co-operate with the pursuit of maintenance or participate in mediation, and acceding to non-resident fathers' every preference regarding contact is unlikely therefore to benefit children. In addition, there is little evidence that policies can significantly affect trends in family structure. A more productive approach would be to accept that family change and diversity are here to stay and to recognise that household resources and continuity and quality of care are more important to children than family structure. Hence, adequate and secure incomes for all families with children, together with services to facilitate responsible decisions about divorce (without imposing unwanted delays) and to negotiate equitable post-divorce arrangements (with separate representation for each party) would be more useful aims, and judgements regarding post-divorce arrangements must always be sensitive to the variability of family relationships. Such an approach would be less likely to deter women from leaving violent men or to fail to protect them and their children when they do.

Such an agenda may be optimistic in the present political context. It requires a genuine commitment to children's welfare as a social (as well as a parental) responsibility, and hence to reducing (rather than increasing) the economic dependence of women on men which limits women's ability to protect themselves and their children from violent men. At a broader level, the extent of men's violence to women and children will only be reduced with a commitment to greater gender equality throughout all areas of society (including the increased involvement of men in parenting pre- as well as post-divorce), more flexible constructions of gender roles (based more on similarity than on difference) and a societal commitment to 'zero tolerance', with effective sanctions against violent men, and accessible alternatives to living with them for women and their children.

Notes

1. Lesbian partnerships are also affected by the Children Act 1989 (under which it is now possible for a female co-parent to acquire parental responsibility for a child

whose mother she lives with) and the Child Support Act (under which lesbian mothers who have lost custody of their children may be required to pay maintenance as absent parents, and lesbian mothers with care of their children who have conceived by artificial insemination by a donor (AID) are required to co-operate with the pursuit of donors for maintenance (if known)).

2. Under existing law (the Divorce Reform Act 1969), irretrievable breakdown is the sole ground for divorce, but the facts by which it can be proved include three 'fault' grounds (adultery, desertion and unreasonable behaviour) and two separation grounds (two years if both parties agree to the divorce, five years if one does not). The majority of divorce petitions are based on fault grounds.

3. Bradshaw and Millar (1991) found an association between maintenance and contact: absent parents with contact were more likely to be paying maintenance. Seltzer (1991) in the United States found that three aspects of fathers' involvement – maintenance, contact and participation in parental decision making – were positively correlated.

4. See *Mediation Quarterly*, Special Issue: *Mediation and Spouse Abuse*, vol. 7, no. 4 (Summer 1990), for discussion.

5. Child Poverty Action Group (CPAG) (1994) note that in the first ten months of the CSA's operation more than half of the 25,000 cases accepted for exemption were accepted for reasons other than 'harm or undue distress' (1994: 65).

6. CPAG (1994) note that 32,600 MAFs were withdrawn in the first nine months of the operation of the CSA, believed to be mostly people who withdrew from benefit altogether. While Peter Lilley argued that these were mostly fraudulent claims, voluntary organisations have argued that this is extremely unlikely. CPAG suggest the reasons are more likely to be reconciliation, employment or the desire to avoid maintenance where the exemption was either not understood or not trusted to cover the lone mother's concern.

7. Agreements for the parent with care to stay in the 'matrimonial home' in return for low or no maintenance have been common in the past but are no longer possible under the Child Support Act.

8. CPAG (1994) have estimated that under a voluntary system approximately 15 per cent of parents with care might not apply.

9. See Hooper (1994) for a review of research on the impact of divorce on children.

11 *Women and private welfare*

Margaret May and Edward Brunsdon

Introduction

In spite of a burgeoning in products and services in the last fifteen years, the private welfare sector in Britain remains a much neglected area of policy research. The process and consequences of privatisation are well documented and there have been several studies of particular forms of private provision, but, as yet, there has been no attempt to draw together its varying forms or to consider the general position of women as consumers *and* producers of private welfare. This chapter addresses these oversights. Drawing on documentary sources, its primary focus is developing an empirical understanding of women's roles in private welfare. It differentiates the main forms of provision and traces recent market trends. At a more conceptual level, it is concerned with identifying key issues that private welfare poses for policy and especially feminist policy research.

Differentiating private welfare

From the outset it is important to recognise that 'private welfare' refers to a wide-ranging and heterogeneous set of options.[1] Trading in welfare products and services can take many forms and occurs in a range of 'markets' with diverse producers and consumers. Provident and for-profit enterprises compete to sell private welfare services and can offer these to organisations in the private, voluntary or public sector. Services can be geared to corporate markets, individual consumers or an array of combinations; they can involve proxy (third-party) purchasers and, in some cases, may be purchased with the support of government subsidies or fiscal concessions.

As such complexity indicates, private welfare's mixed and multiple forms can be represented in various ways. Taking the consumer's perspective as a starting point, however, three criteria suggest themselves as means of differentiation. These are: accessibility, choice and the types of product and service offered. Discriminating by degree, these criteria produce two main types of private welfare: 'employer-sponsored' (or occupationally based) and 'commercial' provision. As its title suggests, employer-sponsored welfare is that purchased on behalf of employees. In large part, what is purchased is framed by organisational or managerial strategies. These act to control accessibility and the range of services offered, and to limit the choices available to end-users. Commercial welfare, by comparison, offers a much wider range of products and services. In this instance, accessibility and choice are dependent on the individual consumer's purchasing power.

Commercial welfare can be 'indirectly' or 'directly' purchased. Indirectly purchased services are primarily insurance-based, the individual procuring 'cover' against one or more of a range of life cycle or other contingencies. This protection can be bought through a diverse range of enterprises, but provision has long been dominated by large financial conglomerates offering services to the public themselves and/or through other agencies. Directly purchased provision comprises a variety of care and support services. With the exception of hospital treatment, these typically function as 'cottage industries' with small local enterprises supplying individual consumers.

Employer-sponsored welfare

Though still marginalised in the policy literature, the benefits and services accruing to employees over and above their pay constitute a major form of private welfare.[2] In many respects employer-sponsored welfare mirrors statutory provision, encompassing financial assistance (in cash and kind), social and health care services, education, training, leisure and community-orientated programmes (May and Brunsdon, 1994). Much of this was traditionally male-orientated and it is only recently that employers have begun to adjust provision to accommodate the work patterns and needs of female employees.

The gendered character of provision remains most visible in the patterning of financial benefits encompassing medical and dental insurance, housing, education, travel and entertainment assistance, occupational sick pay and pensions. The last is arguably the most significant form of employer-sponsored social security and that most subsidised by government. With up to 100,000 schemes, differing in structure, employer control and the degree of inflation-proofing, generalisation is obviously difficult. None the less, it is clear that women's independent access is restricted.

Four factors contribute to this inequity. First of all, British employers are not obliged to offer pension cover (and since 1988 employees are not obliged to join those schemes that are offered). Like other forms of employee welfare, provision is far from universal, being more prevalent in some sectors of the economy than others. Secondly, coverage is more characteristic of large rather than small organisations, especially those with traditionally high levels of unionisation. Though scheme membership grew dramatically in the immediate post-war years, since the late 1960s it has stagnated at just under half the workforce (OPCS, 1993). As a consequence provision is still greater for non-manual workers than for manual workers, and, despite the rhetoric of 'harmonisation', many organisations maintain separate schemes for different levels of personnel. Provision is concentrated in large technology-intensive enterprises, the former public utilities and the public sector, rather than the growth areas of female employment: retailing, catering, tourism and the diffuse small-business sector. Thirdly, like state pensions for which it provides the prototype, occupational provision is still premised on a traditional male model of full-time continuous employment. Pension levels are earnings-related and depend on length of scheme membership (with twenty years' 'service' being widely held as the minimum necessary to secure a 'return'). The majority of schemes exclude part-timers, are conditional on a minimal length of service and, despite efforts to improve 'portability' and conserve pension rights, many still penalise early leavers and those with non-linear or interrupted work patterns (Bone *et al.*, 1992; Davies and Ward, 1992). Finally the schemes, like many other employer benefits, are designed to reward loyalty and organisational position rather than need. The greatest returns accrue to upwardly mobile managers and directors, the elite of whom receive 'top-deck' pensions.

The asymmetry between the patterning of occupational pensions and women's work experiences should be clear to anyone familiar with female employment in Britain and, as recent research shows, impacts on women workers, ex-workers and retirees. Irrespective of women's marital status, pension scheme membership rates reveal a 'stark gender inequality' (Ginn and Arber, 1993) with 46 per cent of men compared to only 24 per cent of women being members. Among employees between the ages of 20 and 59, 39 per cent of women are members compared to 66 per cent of men, with women's membership diverging sharply from men's from their mid-twenties (Ginn and Arber, 1994).

Women are less likely to access the top executive schemes, more likely to be excluded from general schemes because of their part-time status and to lose entitlements through breaks in their working lives. Actuarial practices also allocate women lower annuities than men for the same contributions. Along with women's lower wages, these factors result in less than one in three women compared to two in three men receiving an occupational pension. (Bone *et al.*, 1992; Ginn, 1993). Overall, women's pensions are half those of men's. Yet their work effort and tax contributions still indirectly subsidise the (mainly) male membership. Whilst detailed data on the experiences of ethnic minority women are not available, their employment patterns suggest an even starker discrepancy. Afro-Caribbean women in particular tend to work full- rather than part-time but their position in Britain's occupational and industrial hierarchies is likely to exclude them from this key employee benefit.

For most married women, occupational cover is still conditional on a husband's membership of a pension scheme. The same familialism underpins survivors' benefits (Groves, 1992), although widows' rights remain 'patchy', especially among elderly people (Ginn, 1993). Rising male unemployment, early retirement and escalating divorce rates have re-affirmed the individualist and discretionary nature of employer-based social security and, thereby, the need for women's independent access. Despite the many reform suggestions, divorcees have no recourse to their ex-partner's oc-cupational pension. This could well threaten poverty in retirement for many women (Joshi and Davies, 1991a).

Women's access to other forms of employer financial assistance is similarly limited. For example, fewer women than men are members of occupational sick-pay schemes, which again are less prevalent in those industries where women are concentrated. These schemes vary between manual and non-manual workers (and within the latter) and often exclude part-timers (Dean and Taylor-Gooby, 1990; IDS, 1991a). Women's access to other employee benefits, however, is a reflection less of horizontal than of vertical occupational segregation. Employer-funded medical insurance typ-ically covers only senior management (Bosanquet *et al.*, 1989; IDS, 1993) and until recently was confined to the private sector. Prolonged disability and critical illness insurance are predominantly managerial benefits (Law, 1992), as is housing assistance (Doogan, 1993). Whilst the few women in senior management can access these, most women are again dependent on their partner's occupational status. The wide variety of activities covered by 'corporate entertainment' exhibit a similar pattern, as do the company car and its associated subsidies. Women at the appropriate level in the organisational hierarchy are, like their male colleagues, eligible for this uniquely British perk. However, as the value of the car correlates with company position, few women benefit and those that do tend to receive lower-status vehicles.

The available evidence thus suggests employer-sponsored benefits remain heavily geared to recruiting and retaining a mainly male managerial elite whilst at the same time segmenting the more privileged female employees from both other workers and, of course, those not in paid employment. There are, however, some signs of change, particularly among large employers. The prospect of 'Europeanisation' has prompted occupational pension provision for female part-timers, 17 per cent of whom were scheme members by 1991, compared to 11 per cent in 1987 (OPCS, 1993), though many employers offer money purchase rather than the more beneficial final-salary schemes. European pressure reinforced by the Barber Ruling has also led employers to equalise retirement ages, the majority at 65, a somewhat dubious benefit for women.

Not all forms of financial assistance, however, are vertically segregated and, as a consequence, some are much less gendered. Subsidised cafeterias, meal vouchers and assistance with travel costs (albeit through loans or free parking) are more generally available. Other forms of employer-sponsored welfare also offer more general access. The last decade has seen a significant upsurge in workplace social and health care, with employers funding social work interventions for troubled employees and a profusion of health prevention and promotion initiatives (May and Brunsdon, 1994). These are open to all employees, including part-timers, and often extend to specialist services for female staff, such as cervical and breast cancer screening, other 'well woman' services and counselling on relationship issues which in some companies includes parentcraft.

European Union, demographic and trade union pressures are also impelling improvements in the one occupational benefit exclusive to women, maternity provision (IDS, 1991b). In advance of European requirements some large employers, particularly in the public sector, have improved maternity, paternity and parental leave and contractual maternity pay. Currently, some 14 per cent of women receive contractual maternity pay. The growing availability of such support has contributed to a sharp increase in the number of mothers returning to work within a year of a child's birth, thereby halting women's downward occupational mobility particularly among professional public sector employees (McRae, 1991, 1994).

Some organisations are also developing other services geared to the needs of women in paid employment. The 'family-friendly firm' has been widely canvassed in the human resource management press. Employer-sponsored workplace nurseries, child care vouchers or allowances for pre-school, after-school and school holiday care have been strenuously advocated. As yet however, only 1 per cent of women with under-fives use workplace nurseries and the take-up of places is predominantly in the south-east of England (Holterman and Clark, 1992). A further 1 per cent receive some financial support (OPCS, 1993). A more common (and cheaper) development is the provision of referral services linking working parents with child-minders and other agencies. Other forms of employer-sponsored dependent care are still at an embryonic stage, with provision concentrated on referral and counselling services for carers, a policy endorsed by the government (DoH, 1993).

At an organisational level, the main drive of the family-friendly initiative has been in creating career breaks and offering flexible working arrangements rather than financial support. Despite the terminology of 'working parents/carers' there is still an implicit assumption that caring is a female responsibility that employers accommodate; it is not yet seen as warranting more fundamental changes in *all* employee's work patterns. Where corporate dispensation is offered, it has tended to benefit the minority of 'high-flyers' rather than meet the needs of the mass of female employees. In many ways this has amplified divisions among women (Truman, 1992; Buswell and Jenkins, 1994).

Commercial welfare: 'indirect' services and products

Indirect commercial welfare encompasses a range of insurance products which have mushroomed in tandem with the decline in the value of state benefits over the last fifteen years. Though national data are not available, the gender profile of consumers in these markets can be inferred from three key insurance packages: private pensions, medical insurance and long-term care.

Given their employment patterns and the limits of occupational schemes, for many women the most important welfare product offered by the commercial market is a private pension. For the self-employed it is the only option. Large-scale consumption, however, is a very recent development and was triggered by the 1986 Social Security Act. This gave employees paying national insurance contributions the option of purchasing 'appropriate personal pension plans' with a fiscal incentive to do so. In advocating personal pensions, the government's supporters emphasised the scheme's potential for reducing public expenditure and enhancing freedom of choice. It was seen as a way of reducing reliance on employer-determined welfare (Waine, 1992) and encouraging personal providence and self-responsibility. Personal pensions were also construed as filling the gaps in pension coverage. This, along with government subsidies, quickly featured in personal pensions marketing, much of which was targeted at women.

By 1989 over a hundred financial institutions had responded to this new state-sponsored market (Blake, 1992), with building societies, banks, insurance companies and unit trust enterprises vying for customers and deploying the full repertoire of modern advertising to sell mostly defined-contribution or money purchase schemes. By 1993, over 5 million individuals were buying personal pensions, confounding government projections and at a cost to the Treasury of some £7 billion (Hughes and Hunter, 1993). General Household Survey (GHS) data, collected for the first time in 1991, show 26 per cent of male compared to 19 per cent of female full-time employees and 11 per cent of female part-timers were members of personal pension schemes. Among the self-employed, for whom personal pensions are even more critical, 66 per cent of full-time self-employed males, compared to 42 per cent of full-time and 20 per cent of part-time self-employed women were members (OPCS, 1993). Not surprisingly, the purchasers appear to be drawn particularly from those occupational groups and organisations where employer benefits are less prevalent.

Despite their portability and other apparent attractions for women, personal pensions raise a number of issues (Davies and Ward, 1992; Carr, 1993). For married women dependent on a spouse's purchase, personal pensions, unlike most employers' schemes, do not automatically incorporate dependant benefits. For women buying their own retirement cover, other issues arise. To begin with, the transaction costs of personal pensions generate high premiums, with the greater costs falling disproportionately on those purchasing the lowest pensions. The premiums themselves are also often beyond the means of the low-waged and those with irregular employment. What is more, any scheme based on earnings over a lifetime implies a lower retirement income for women, whilst the early contributions necessary to produce the best returns in money purchase schemes are nullified by women's interrupted work patterns. Finally, the returns and the annuities they purchase are contingent on the performance of the chosen scheme and the vagaries of the financial markets. Up to the 1989 Finances Act, the categories of eligible securities available for investment were mainly restricted to UK-quoted shares and investment trusts. But it has since been possible to invest in overseas shares, unquoted UK trusts, unit trusts, gilt and commercial property.

Choosing a personal pension thus demands a close 'reading' of market trends and skilled advice. Yet, as recent inquiries have shown, the commission-driven sales of personal pensions by financial institutions has led to large-scale 'mis-selling'. Large numbers of those least likely to benefit, particularly women, have been persuaded to leave their current schemes. Recent estimates suggest that over 250,000 women have been disadvantaged by abandoning SERPS. Ninety per cent of those exiting employer schemes, including many nurses, teachers and care workers, have been equally mis-advised, buying insecurity rather than a provident old age (Hughes and Hunter, 1993). Compensation has been promised, a Securities Investment Board inquiry is under way and the regulatory bodies have, belatedly, taken action. The debacle may, as personal pensions' supporters contend, prove to be a 'growing pain' (Bell, 1994). But it has, like the Maxwell occupational pension scandal, thrown into sharp relief the limitations of current regulatory mechanisms and the uncertainties of self-provision. In the meantime, the commercial market remains ill adjusted to women's pension needs.

Other types of commercial welfare insurance such as the proliferating income and critical illness packages and, most notably, private medical insurance (PMI) also seem similarly ill adjusted to women's needs. From the consumers' perspective PMI is purchased in one of three ways: independently, through an employer scheme, or through a group scheme where companies, professional bodies or unions act as 'umbrellas' but employees pay the premiums. After a slow, uneven growth from 1.2 per cent of the UK population in 1955 to 5 per cent in 1979, the numbers insured escalated to 12.2 per cent of the population in 1991 (Laing, 1992). The upsurge was driven primarily by increased company purchasing, but predictions of coverage extending to 20 per cent of the population have been stalled by the recession. The drop in company-paid subscribers in 1991 was offset by an equivalent (3 per cent) rise in personal purchasing, highlighting the extent to which PMI has also been consumer-driven (Laing, 1992, 1993a). Individual purchase has also been spurred by the development of high-street retailing through banks and building societies. Purchase by the over-sixties was given an extra incentive by tax concessions in the 1990 budget. This appears, however, to have triggered a shift between schemes rather than an overall increase in the numbers of retirees insured.

Of the twenty-eight private medical insurers in the United Kingdom, the brand leaders are the provident associations: BUPA, PPP and WPA. They now face stiff competition from commercial operators whose market share grew from 9 per cent in 1985 to 14 per cent by 1991 (Laing,1992). Traditionally, PMI offerings were limited to minor elective surgery. Product design remains remarkably conservative but the impetus of commercial ventures has led to some widening, and offers now include GP minor surgery, maternity, home and hospice care, single-organ or single-illness insurance and, most notably, low-cost policies aimed at Hospital Trust pay beds and dental insurance where the demise of NHS dentistry has created a 'new market' (Fitzhugh, 1993).

Though the socio-economic profile of PMI consumers is clear, research into the reasons for purchase and its gender and ethnic divisions is limited (Calnan *et al.*,

1993). GHS data showed purchasing was highest among professional workers (34 per cent in 1987), declining sharply (to 2 per cent) among unskilled manual workers. Geographically, consumers were concentrated in the affluent south-east (OPCS, 1989). The industry has attempted to broaden its customer base, developing 'waiting-list policies' and 'family packages' aimed at white-collar and skilled manual groups and appealing to traditional familialist assumptions. Though the first 'single-illness products' were for private treatment of breast and cervical cancer, women generally have not been seen as independent purchasers.

Despite efforts to diversify, PMI remains a 'luxury purchase' (Laing, 1992). The typical policy-holders are white middle-aged men in managerial or professional occupations. The limited evidence available suggests PMI is rarely accessed by Britain's ethnic minorities. Employer purchase is highly selective, geared to minimising work disruptions and securing the commitment of senior executives. High status within the organisation also secures 'family cover', though many schemes entail employee funding of such 'extras'. The 1987 GHS revealed 11 per cent of married men held policies, compared to 2 per cent of married women, but 10 per cent of married women were covered by their partners' insurance (OPCS, 1989). Four per cent of single women, compared to 7 per cent of single men were policy holders. Like their married counterparts, single insured women's economic position differs sharply from that of most women.

A similar double segmentation appears to characterise emergent forms of insurance, such as dread disease and long-term care insurance (LTCI). The latter potentially offers women, with their greater longevity, considerable benefit. In Britain, it is a very recent innovation. The first products were launched in 1991 and two versions are on offer, appealing to different clientele: pre-funded schemes (LTCI, LTCI linked to pensions or life insurance) and immediate care products (annuities, equity release). With an ageing population a high demand might be anticipated, but British and American research suggests that, initially, the market is likely to be confined to the newly retired and those approaching retirement (Laing, 1991, 1993b). An estimated 20 per cent of retirees are considered to have sufficient resources to purchase LTCI and it is to this 'safari market' that current sales are geared. The government's brake on state support, the decline in NHS long-stay beds and the likely need for care imply a larger future market for pre-funded schemes. However, public awareness of the need for cover is, as yet, limited. Significantly, gender does not appear to feature in the market's profiling, women being subsumed within a (male-led) household and not, in the first instance, perceived as likely purchasers in their own right. For the majority of women, LTC insurance, like much commercial welfare, is thus a function of marriage rather than women's independent earning power.

Commercial welfare: 'direct services' and products

Directly purchased commercial welfare appears to offer women more opportunities than its indirect counterpart. These services, however, are also stratified both between men and women and among women, as an examination of private hospitals, residential, domiciliary and child care reveals.

Like PMI, private acute hospital provision has expanded, albeit unevenly, from 150 hospitals with 6,671 beds in 1979 to 220 hospitals with 11,414 beds by 1993 (Laing, 1991; Fitzhugh, 1993). Much of this growth is due to an influx of for-profit operators. Capitalising on the deregulation of the health market by the Thatcher governments (Mohan, 1991) the for-profit market share increased from 41 per cent of private beds in 1979 to 60 per cent in 1990 (Laing, 1992). Increased pay-bed authorisations in the 1980s and the establishment of NHS Hospital Trusts have added further complexity to the market, many seeking to increase their revenues through new style private wings and pay beds. Information on these is no longer collected nationally. Recent estimates, however, suggest that hospitals have increased their income from selling amenity beds and other 'extras' by 45 per cent during the first two years of the internal market (Brindle, 1994). NHS providers now hold some 11.2 per cent (worth £135 million) of the market (Laing, 1992), although they betray the same regional imbalances as private hospitals.

In terms of treatment, private hospitals focus on high-volume, acute elective surgery. On average they command a fifth of such operations, rising to nearly a third in some parts of the south-east (Nicholl *et al.*, 1989). A significant proportion are geared to women's health care. Along with ophthalmic and general surgery, they conducted 28 per cent of hip replacements and 24 per cent of hysterectomies in 1992 (Fitzhugh, 1993) and the majority of abortions (56 per cent in 1990). Sterilisation and infertility treatment, where the NHS provision is again limited, are also predominantly supplied by the private sector (Laing, 1992).

As several studies have indicated, women use private hospitals more than men, which reflects their higher usage of health care services generally. A third of patients are fee-paying and it is estimated that the majority of these are older women (Propper and Maynard, 1989; Laing, 1993b). The other two-thirds are funded by insurance. Women again predominate, although, ironically, this is generally accessed through their partners' PMI (Higgins, 1988; Nicholl *et al.*, 1989). The unusual gendering of private hospital provision, however, has attracted little research attention. Available evidence suggests that women, like men, use the service pragmatically to avoid the perceived problems of the NHS and to capitalise on employer-purchased insurance. However, within this, there are different sets of calculations. Wiles (1993) suggests that women's take-up, unlike men's, is structured by their caring roles. As paying customers, they also feel they have more control over their treatment and greater privacy. Thorogood's study (1992) of Afro-Caribbean, working-class women reveals a similar calculation. For these women, a private GP consultation offers not only a more personalised and speedier service but a sense of control, which itself appears to redress racial, class and gender inequalities.

Whereas private medical treatment offers some women greater consumer sovereignty, other forms of direct commercial provision, like the long-term home care sector, present a more complex picture. The nursing and residential home industry has seen a meteoric growth, and by 1990 for-profit capacity exceeded that offered by

Table 11.1 Nursing and residential home places 1970–90

| Date | Residential home places | | | Nursing home places | |
	Local authority	Private	Voluntary	Private/voluntary	
1970	108,700	23,700	40,100	20,300	
1980	134,500	37,400	42,600	26,900	
				Private	Voluntary
1990	125,600	155,600	40,000	112,600	10,500

Source: after Laing (1992)

the statutory and voluntary sectors (see Table 11.1). Most of this was taken up by elderly widows (Laing, 1991). Their admission was facilitated by what was tantamount to a public voucher system funded through social security bed-and-lodging payments. Between 1979 and 1992 state contributions to care homes rose 250-fold (from £10 million to £2,530 million), the major beneficiaries being private homes. This upsurge in social security support was paralleled by an increase in both self-funding and top-up payments by users or their relatives, especially in nursing homes. Overall, some 40 per cent of customers were self-paying. With top-ups, two-thirds of care home revenue came from private sources, most of it from assets released from the sale of housing. Although the property slump of 1990/2 affected this trend, prompting a 'remarkable ballooning' in the number of residents claiming income support (48–70 per cent), it has now been effectively counter-balanced by the full implementation of the 1990 NHS and Community Care Act's funding changes and private payments for long-term care are likely to rise again.

Admission to long-term care, for most residents, has been more a product of family 'crisis' than pre-planning. Evidence suggests that decisions are taken primarily by women relatives and based on local 'knowledge', owners' policies and available vacancies rather than informed market preference (Challis and Bartlett, 1987; J. Phillips, 1992). Recent community care changes could have led to more informed consumption; however, early indicators suggest that the ability to choose will vary with the source of funding. For those dependent on public support, much will hinge on the flexibility of local authority purchasing styles. Self- or partial funders retain choice, especially if they by-pass local authority needs assessments and enter directly. The potential for such queue-jumping raises fears of an emerging two-tier provision, both among and within homes, in which self- or partial funders take up the better accommodation.

At one level, the long-term care industry epitomises the conception of the welfare market advocated by neo-liberal writers. It consists of a mass of small competing enterprises operated by owner-managers. The majority are 'corner shop' style ventures (Hatchett, 1990). At another level it is very different in that the industry is dominated by women, trading jointly with their husbands or singly and employing a mainly female labour force selling to a largely female clientele. In entering this market, during the 1980s, female entrepreneurs clearly sought a profitable return from a promising, government-subsidised, business niche. Financial gain, however, has not been the sole motivation (Todd, 1990; J. Phillips, 1992). For those 'displaced' by public sector restructuring it has been an alternative career path, a factor that also applied to the many small hoteliers who converted their establishments in the early 1980s. More significantly, for the many former social and health care workers, self-employment offered an alternative to blocked career structures and the perceived bureaucracy of the public care sector. It also offered an opportunity to combine entrepreneurial initiatives with their professional skills and domestic responsibilities.

Whatever the motivation, owner-management has not automatically provided women with a route to independence or more client-centred caring. Most homes operate on tight financial margins, the main (and unstable) asset being the property's capital value rather than earned income. Where women are involved in joint ventures with their husbands, it appears that many replicate the traditional sexual division of labour. Husbands take responsibility for 'external' management, wives for internal supervision and direct care-giving. This orthodoxy is also reflected in the invocation of familial terminology. Long-term care homes rely heavily on the client appeal of the 'family business'. The label and promise of 'a family atmosphere' not only reconcile the potential conflict between caring and trading in welfare, they also facilitate labour discipline in an area dependent on personal service for low pay and disguise tensions between producers and consumes.

Similar tensions characterise the other main forms of 'direct' commercial welfare, namely domiciliary and child care. Very little is known about domiciliary care (Sinclair *et al.*, 1990), primarily because it takes the form of self-employed female labour purveying domestic and care skills on a cash basis often outside the formal economy. For these vendors, employment both resolves and re-affirms their second-ary labour market position, enabling them to accommodate work to domestic commit-ments by selling 'female' competences at the levels their predominantly female clients can afford. The fragmented and labour-intensive nature of this industry has, as yet, restrained corporate intervention. Localised small businesses akin to long-term care homes and concentrating on intensive care for elderly people and people with dis-abilities are, however, emerging, partly stimulated by the Independent Living Fund. Again, former public sector female employees working from home, and often drawing on past colleagues, appear to be the prime movers (Midwinter, 1986).

Private child care also involves diverse providers. Whilst still a secondary form to informal care provision, paid care grew sharply in the 1980s. By 1991 one-fifth of working mothers and nearly one-half of those with children under five relied on bought care, the heaviest users being women in professional jobs (Marsh and McKay, 1993a). Provision itself is segmented between agency-organised nanny and *au pair* care, small localised, mainly female-headed businesses offering 'nursery' care for pre-school children, self-employed nannies and the predominant service mode, registered child-minders. Though child-minding has lost its earlier negative image, pay remains low and the market generally is unlikely to alter whilst many female consumers remain concentrated at the lower, insecure end of the labour market (Joshi and Davies, 1993).

' *Issues arising*

Tracing the composition and distribution of employer-sponsored and commercial welfare raises key concerns for policy and feminist policy research. The most immediate and, perhaps, most obvious is the need to redress the neglect of private welfare in the literature. There is a clear requirement for detailed empirical research on the plurality of its markets, market participants and their grounds for participation. The complex gendering of private welfare and women's roles as both producers and consumers must form a central axis of such investigations if the current shifts in Britain's welfare mix are to be fully assessed.

Within this general remit, there are several clusters of issues worthy of individual attention. The first concerns the extent to which some forms of private welfare depend on female production *and* consumption and the way this impacts on market operations. Long-term, domiciliary and child care in particular are heavily dependent on female enterprise, trade in traditional female skills and operate with relatively low capital, low labour costs and tight profit margins. The dynamics of such female producer–consumer relations warrant further research, as do labour relations in these industries. It is clear, however, that though women are pre-eminent in these markets, production and consumption are still set by the wider sexual division of labour. The low material rewards to producers seem to be the direct consequence of the value accorded caring and the limited purchasing power of their mainly female consumers. Yet for many women this is the only way to enter the market as producers or to gain employment.

Women's propensity to buy private welfare services raises a second cluster of issues. Of particular importance are the grounds for women's purchase. For instance, are some women buying welfare as a means of redressing the gender imbalances created and sustained by public welfare services? Equally significant is the extent to which private welfare markets create divisions not simply between men and women, but among women as well. A minority of women, predominantly White and cushioned by managerial or professional occupations, can purchase a range of welfare products. They are also likely to benefit from employer-sponsored provision and can still access statutory, voluntary and informal resources. In comparison, the majority of women appear 'welfare poor'. Though this can be mediated by marital status and partners' occupations, private welfare clearly individuates and divides women from each other.

Differences between women, whether as consumers or producers, would clearly be obfuscated if research was focused solely on gendered relations. This should not detract, however, from female–male divisions so much as add a further dimension to analyses: gender divisions remain central to an understanding of women's position within the welfare marketplace. By comparison with their male counterparts, women generally have less financial autonomy. As workers they earn less and their spending power is still constrained by domestic and caring responsibilities. Their consumer sovereignty and choice are consequently limited. It is also the case that for many women private welfare is accessible only through dependence on a male partner.

The third and final cluster of issues operates at a more theoretical level and centres on the need to reconceptualise the view of the market that currently underwrites much of the discussion of private welfare. Developed by Hayek and deployed by advocates of private markets, this essentialist conception describes 'the' market as a form of social co-ordination of voluntary economic exchange. Individual buyers and sellers, possessing different amounts of knowledge of consumer preferences, pursue their own economic interests through the exchange of goods and services (Hindess, 1987).

Following orthodox neo-classical economics, Hayek treats this conception as an entity that can be understood independently of both the institutional framework in which it is embedded and the calculations of participating agents (Tomlinson, 1990). Abstracting 'market' from its institutional settings and the calculations of agents in this way allows Hayek to operate with the twin notions of a 'natural' family and a 'natural' sexual division of labour and, further, to treat them as given. By taking them for granted, he and his followers have effectively ignored 'the space women inhabit' (Pascall, 1986). They therefore fail to acknowledge both the extent to which women participate in private welfare markets and, when compared with men, the social and economic conditions of their participation. Ironically, this marginalisation has been compounded by Hayek's many opponents, who in their efforts to defend state provision have left unquestioned what is effectively a gendered conception of 'the' market.

Bringing women in would reveal the obstacles to both their industrial citizenship and consumer opportunities. It would also encourage a rethinking of current market conceptions by forcing analysts to take account of the plurality of welfare markets, their diverse constituents, conditions of operation and participants. This is particularly pertinent in the light of the current government's exhortations in favour of private welfare. While ostensibly designed to maximise individual freedom, they are frequently packaged with an espousal of family responsibility. The implications for women are far-reaching. Without a radical degendering of both paid and unpaid work, greater reliance on private welfare in current circumstances will entail greater dependency on men.

Notes

1. The focus here is on social protection, health and social care. Housing is discussed elsewhere in this volume (Chapter 5) and also by Gilroy (1994).
2. Other forms of employment-related welfare provided by trade unions and professional associations will not be discussed here, though many unions seem to be shifting to this service role (Heery and Kelly, 1994).

References

Abbott, P. and Wallace, C. (1990), *An Introduction to Sociology: Feminist perspectives*, London: Routledge.

Acker, S. (1992a), 'Gender, collegiality and teachers' workplace culture in Britain: in search of the women's culture', paper presented to the American Educational Research Association, New Orleans.

Acker, S. (1992b), 'Creating careers: women teachers at work', *Curriculum Enquiry*, 22, 2: 141–63.

Adler, M., Arnott, M., *et al.* (1994), 'Scottish experiences of devolved management: an enhanced role for school boards', paper presented to the CEDAR International Conference, Changing Educational Structures: Policy and Practice, University of Warwick.

Adler, M., Petch, A. and Tweedie, J. (1989), *Parental Choice and Educational Policy*, Edinburgh: Edinburgh University Press.

Afshar, H. and Maynard, M. (eds) (1994), *The Dynamics of 'Race' and Gender: Some feminist interventions*, London: Taylor & Francis.

Age Concern England (1993), *No Time to Lose: First impressions of the community care reforms*, London: ACE.

Ahrentzen, S. and Franck, K. (eds) (1989), *New Households, New Housing*, New York: Van Nostrand Reinhold.

Aitken-Swan, J. (1977), *Fertility Control and the Medical Profession*, London: Croom Helm.

Akeroyd, A. (1994), 'Gender, race and ethnicity in official statistics', in H. Afshar and M. Maynard (eds) (1994), *The Dynamics of 'Race' and Gender: Some feminist interventions*, London: Taylor & Francis.

Alber, J. (1993), 'Health and social services', in A. Walker, J. Alber and A.M. Guillemard,

Older People in Europe: Social and economic policies, Brussels: Commission of the European Communities.

Amin, K. with Oppenheim, C. (1992), *Poverty in Black and White: Deprivation and ethnic minorities*, London: Child Poverty Action Group and the Runnymede Trust.

Amos, V. and Parmar, P. (1984), 'Challenging imperial feminism', *Feminist Review*, 17: 3–19.

Andrews, B. (1994), 'Family violence in a social context: factors relating to male abuse of children', in J. Archer (ed.), *Male Violence*, London: Routledge.

Anlin, S. (1989), *Out but not Down: The housing needs of lesbians*, London: Homeless Action.

Anthias, F. (1990), 'Race and class revisited: conceptualising race and racisms', *Sociological Review*, 38, 1 (February): 19–42.

Anthias, F. and Yuval-Davis, N. (1983), 'Contextualising feminism: ethnic gender and class divisions', *Feminist Review*, 15: 162–75.

Anthias, F. and Yuval-Davis, N. (1992), *Racialised Boundaries: Race, nation, gender, colour and class and the anti-racist struggle*, London: Routledge.

Arber, S. and Ginn, J. (1990), 'The meaning of informal care: gender and the contribution of elderly people', *Ageing and Society*, 10: 429–54.

Arber, S. and Ginn, J. (1991), *Gender and Later Life: A sociological analysis of resources and constraints*, London: Sage.

Arber, S. and Ginn, J. (1992), 'Class and caring: a forgotten dimension', *Sociology*, 26, 4: 619–34.

Arber, S., Gilbert, N. and Evandrou, M. (1988), 'Gender, household composition and receipt of domiciliary services by elderly disabled people', *Journal of Social Policy*, 17, 2: 153–75.

Arnot, M. (1985), *Race and Gender: Equal opportunities policies in education*, Oxford: Pergamon.

Arnot, M. and Weiler, K. (1993), *Feminism and Social Justice in Education*, London: Falmer Press.

Arnot, M. and Weiner, G. (eds) (1987), *Gender and the Politics of Schooling*, London: Hutchinson.

Aronson, J. (1990), 'Women's perspectives on informal care of the elderly: public ideology and personal experience of giving and receiving care', *Ageing and Society*, 10: 61–84.

Association for Improvements in Maternity Services (AIMS) (1991), Supplementary Memorandum submitted by AIMS in *House of Commons Health Committee Second Report*, Vol. II, Minutes of Evidence, London: HMSO, pp. 471–99.

Atkin, K. (1991), 'Community care in a multi-racial society: incorporating the user view', *Policy and Politics*, 19, 3, 159–66.

Atkin, K. (1992), 'Similarities and differences between informal carers', in J. Twigg (ed.), *Carers: Research and practice*, London: HMSO.

Audit Commission (1986), *Making a Reality of Community Care*, London: HMSO.

Audit Commission (1994), *A Prescription for Improvement*, London: HMSO.

Aziz, R. (1992), 'Feminism and the challenge of racism: deviance or difference?', in H. Crowley and S. Himmelweit (eds) *Knowing Women: Feminism and knowledge*, Cambridge: Polity Press.

Baginsky, M., Baker, L., *et al.* (1991), *Towards Effective Partnerships in School Governance*, Slough: National Foundation for Educational Research.

Balbo, L. (1987), 'Crazy quilts: rethinking the welfare state debate from a women's point of view', in A. Showstack Sassoon (ed.) (1987), *Women and the State*, London: Hutchinson.

Baldock, J. (1994), 'The personal social services: the politics of care', in V. George and S. Miller (eds), *Social Policy towards 2000: Squaring the welfare circle*, London: Routledge.

Baldock, J. and Evers, A. (1992), 'Innovations and care of the elderly: the cutting edge of change for social welfare systems. Examples from Sweden, the Netherlands and the United Kingdom', *Ageing and Society*, 12: 289–312.

Baldock, J. and Ungerson, C. (1993), 'Consumer perceptions of an emerging mixed economy of care', in A. Evers and I. Svetlik (eds), *Balancing Pluralism: New welfare mixes in care for the elderly*, Aldershot: Avebury.

Barker, M. (1981), *The New Racism*, London: Junction.

Barrett, M. and Phillips, A. (eds) (1992), *Destabilising Theory: Contemporary feminist debates*, Cambridge: Polity Press.

Barron, J. (1990), *Not Worth the Paper . . .? The effectiveness of legal protection for women and children experiencing domestic violence*, Bristol: WAFE.

Bartholomew, R., Hibbett, A. and Sidaway, J. (1992), 'Lone parents and the labour market: evidence from the Labour Force Survey', *Employment Gazette* (November): 559–78.

Begum, N. (1990), *Burden of Gratitude: Women with disabilities receiving personal care*, Warwick: University of Warwick, Social Care Practice Centre.

Bell, M. (1994), 'Privatizing pensions', in M. Bell, E. Butler, D. Marsland and M. Pirie (eds), *The End of the Welfare State*, London: Adam Smith Institute.

Beuret, K. (1991), 'Women and transport', in M. Maclean and D. Groves (eds), *Women's Issues in Social Policy*, London: Routledge.

Beveridge, W. (1942), *Social Insurance and Allied Services*, Cmnd 6404, London: HMSO.

Bhat, A., Carr-Hill, R. and Ohri, S. (1988), *Britain's Black Population: A new perspective*, The Radical Statistics Race Group, Aldershot: Gower.

Bhavnani, K.K. (1990), 'Is violence masculine?', in S. Grewal *et al.* (eds), *Charting the Journey: Writings by Black and Third World women*, London: Sheba.

Bhavnani, K.K. (1992), 'Talking racism and the editing of women's studies', in D. Richardson and V. Robinson (eds), *Introducing Women's Studies*, London: Macmillan.

Bhavnani, K.K. (1994), 'Tracing the contours: feminist research and feminist objectivity', in H. Afshar and M. Maynard (eds) (1994), *The Dynamics of 'Race' and Gender: Some feminist interventions*, London: Taylor & Francis.

Bhavnani, K.K. and Collins, D. (1993), 'Racism and feminism: an analysis of the Anita Hill and Clarence Thomas hearings', *New Community*, 19, 3 (April): 493–505.

Bhavnani, K.K. and Coulson, M. (1986), 'Transforming socialist feminism: the challenge of racism', *Feminist Review*, 23: 81–92.

Binney, V., Harkell, G. and Nixon, J. (1981), *Leaving Violent Men*, London: WAFE.

Blair, M. (1993), 'Black parents and education reform', paper presented to the International Sociology of Education Conference, Sheffield.

Blake, D. (1992), *Issues in Pension Funding*, London: Routledge.

Blake, J. (1994a), 'Homeless all at sea', *Roof* (May/June): 26–9.

Blake, J. (1994b), 'The agents of change', *Roof* (July/August): 26–9.

Bone, M., Gregory, J., Gill, B. and Lader, D. (1992), *Retirement and Retirement Plans*, Office of Population Censuses and Surveys, London: HMSO.

Borkowski, M., Murch, M. and Walker, V. (1983), *Marital Violence: The community response*, London: Tavistock.

Bosanquet, N., Laing, W. and Propper, C. (1989), *Elderly Consumers in Britain: Europe's poor relation?*, London: Laing & Buisson.

Bottomley, A. (1985), 'What is happening to family law? A feminist critique of conciliation', in J. Brophy and C. Smart (eds), *Women-in-Law*, London: Routledge & Kegan Paul.

Boulard, J.C. (1991), *Vivre ensemble: rapport de la mission parlementaire*, Publication de l'Assemblée Nationale no. 2135, Paris: Assemblée Nationale.

Bowe, R., Ball, J. and Gewirtz, S. (1994), 'Parental choice, consumption and social theory: the operation of micro markets in education', *British Journal of Educational Studies*, 42, 1: 38–52.

Bowker, L. H., Barbittel, M. and McFerrow, J.R. (1988), 'On the relationship between wife beating and child abuse', in K. Yllo and M. Bograd (eds), *Feminist Perspectives on Wife Abuse*, London: Sage.

Bradshaw, J. (1993), *Household Budgets and Living Standards*, York: Joseph Rowntree Foundation.

Bradshaw, J. and Holmes, H. (1989), *Living on the Edge*, Newcastle: Tyneside Child Poverty Action Group.

Bradshaw, J. and Millar, J. (1991), *Lone Parent Families in the UK*, Department of Social Security, Research Report no. 6, London: HMSO.

Brah, A. (1992), 'Difference, diversity and differentiation', in J. Donald and A. Rattansi (eds), *'Race', Culture and Difference*, London: Sage/Open University.

Brah, A. (1994), ' "Race" and "culture" in the gendering of labour markets', in Brent Community Health Council (1981), *Black People and the Health Service*, London: Brent Community Health Council.

Brailey, M. (1985), *Women's Access to Council Housing*, Occasional Paper no. 25, Glasgow: the Planning Exchange.

Brewer, R. M. (1993), 'Theorizing race, class and gender: the new scholarship of Black feminist intellectuals and Black Women's Labour', in M. James and A.P.A. Busia (eds), *Theorizing Black Feminisms: The visionary pragmatism of black women*, New York: Routledge.

Brindle, D. (1994), ' "Hospital extras" raise £150m under market sales system', *The Guardian*, 16 March.

Brion, M. (1987), 'The housing problems women face', *Housing Review*, 36, 4: 139–40.

Broadbent, J. and Laughlin, R. (1993), *The Values of Accountancy and Education: A question of gender?*, Dept of Educational Research Open Seminar Series, Lancaster University.

Broadbent, J., Richard, L., *et al.* (1993), *Financial Controls and Schools: Accounting in 'public' and 'private' spheres*, Sheffield: Sheffield University Management School Discussion Paper Series.

Brook, E. and Davis, A. (eds) (1985), *Women, the Family and Social Work*, London: Tavistock.

Brotchie, J. and Hills, D. (1991), *Equal Shares in Caring*, London: Socialist Health Association.

Brown, C. (1984), *Black and White Britain: The third PSI survey*, London: Heinemann.

Brown, H. and Smith, H. (1993), 'Women caring for people: the mismatch between rhetoric and women's reality?', *Policy and Politics*, 21, 3: 185–93.

Brown, H.C. (1992), 'Lesbians, the state and social work practice', in M. Langan and L. Day (eds), *Women, Oppression and Social Work: Issues in anti-discriminatory practice*, London: Routledge.

Brown, P. (1993), 'Breast cancer: a lethal inheritance', *New Scientist*, 18 September, 34–7.

Brown, S. (1994), 'Educational change and children's progress: some north–south comparisons', plenary address presented to the CEDAR International Conference, University of Warwick.

Brownmiller, S. (1976), *Against our Will: Men, women and rape*, Harmondsworth: Penguin.

Bruegel, I. (1989), 'Sex and race in the labour market', *Feminist Review*, 32: 49–68.

Bruegel, I. (1994), 'Labour market prospects for women from ethnic minorities', in R. Lindley (ed.), *Labour Market Structures and Prospects for Women*, Manchester: Equal Opportunities Commission.

Bryan, B., Dadzie, S. and Scafe, S. (1985), *The Heart of the Race: Black women's lives in Britain*, London: Virago.

Bucher, H. and Schmidt, J. (1993), 'Does routine ultrasound scanning improve outcome in pregnancy? Meta-analysis of various outcome measures', *British Medical Journal*, 307: 13–17.

Bull, J. (1991), *Housing Consequences of Relationship Breakdown*, University of York: SPRU.

Bull, J. (1993), *Housing Consequences of Relationship Breakdown*, Department of the Environment, London: HMSO.

Bulmer, M., Lewis, J. and Piachaud, D. (1989), *The Goals of Social Policy*, London: Unwin Hyman.

Burgoyne, C. (1990), 'Money in marriage: how patterns of allocation both reflect and conceal power', *The Sociological Review*, 38, 4: 634–65.

Burgoyne, C. and Millar, J. (1994), 'Enforcing child support obligations: the attitudes of separated fathers', *Policy and Politics*, 22, 2: 95–104.

Burns, B. and Phillipson, C. (1986), *Drugs, Ageing and Society*, London: Croom Helm.

Buswell, C. and Jenkins, S. (1994), 'Equal opportunities policies, employment and patriarchy', *Gender, Work and Organization*, 1, 2: 83–93.

Byrne, E. (1978), *Women and Education*, London: Tavistock.

Cahill, M. (1991), 'The greening of social policy', in N. Manning (ed.), *Social Policy Review 1990–91*, Harrow: Longman.

Cain, H. and Yuval-Davis, N. (1990), ' "The Equal Opportunities Community" and the anti-racist struggle', *Critical Social Policy* (Autumn): 5–26.

Callan, T., Nolan, B. and Whelan, C. T. (1993), 'Resources, deprivation and the measurement of poverty', *Journal of Social Policy*, 22, 2: 141–72.

Callender, C. (1987), 'Women seeking work', in S. Fineman (ed.), *Unemployment: Personal and social consequences*, London: Tavistock.

Callender, C. (1992), 'Redundancy, unemployment and poverty', in C. Glendinning and J. Millar (eds), *Women and Poverty in Britain: The 1990s*, Hemel Hempstead: Harvester Wheatsheaf.

Callender, C., Court, C., Thompson, M. and Patch, A. (forthcoming), *Employers and Family Credit: Their knowledge, practices and attitudes*, Department of Social Security, Research Report, London: HMSO.

Callender, C., Toye, J., Connor, H. and Spilsbury, M. (1993), *National Vocational Qualifications and Scottish Vocational Qualifications: Early indications of employers' take-up and use*, Brighton: Institute of Manpower Studies.

Calnan, M., Cant, S. and Gabe, J. (1993), *Going Private: Why people pay for their health care*, Buckingham: Open University Press.

Campbell, J.C. (1992), ' "If I can't have you, no one can": power and control in homicide of female partners', in J. Radford and D. Russell (eds), *Femicide: The politics of woman killing*, Buckingham: Open University Press.

Carby, H. (1982), 'White women listen! Black feminism and the boundaries of sisterhood', in Centre for Contemporary Cultural Studies, *The Empire Strikes Back: Race and racism in 70s Britain*, London: Hutchinson.

Carr, M. (1993), 'Women, pensions and the state', *Benefits*, 8: 9–13.

Central Statistical Services (1993), *Regional Trends*, London: HMSO.

Challis, L. and Bartlett, H. (1987), *Old and Ill*, Institute of Gerontology Research Paper no. 1, London: Age Concern.

Child Poverty Action Group (1994), *Putting the Treasury First*, London: CPAG.

Child Support Agency (1994), *Child Support Agency: The first two years*, DSS.

Clarke, J. (ed.) (1993), *A Crisis in Care? Challenges to social work*, London: Sage.

Clarke, J., Cochrane, A. and McLaughlin, E. (eds) (1994), *Managing Social Policy*, London: Sage.

Clarke, K. (1991), *Women and Training: A review*, Manchester: EOC.

Clarke, K., Craig, G. and Glendinning, C. (1993), *Children Come First? The Child Support Act and lone parent families*, Manchester: Barnados, the Children's Society, NCH, NSPCC and SCF.

Clarke, K., Craig, G. and Glendinning, C. (1994), 'Child support, parental responsibility and the law: an examination of the implications of recent British legislation', paper presented to the thirty-first International Sociological Association, Committee on Family Research Seminar, London, 28–30 April.

Cm. 849 (1989), *Caring for People: Community care in the next decade and beyond*, London: HMSO.

Cm. 2563 (1994), *Competitiveness: Helping business to win*, London: HMSO.

Cockburn, C. (1987), *Two-track Training*, London: Macmillan.

Cockburn, C. (1991), *In the Way of Women*, Basingstoke: Macmillan.

Cohen, P. (1992), 'It's racism what dunnit', in J. Donald and A. Rattansi (eds), *'Race', Culture and Difference*, London: Sage/Open University.

Cohen, N. and Weir, S. (1994), 'Welcome to Quangoland', *Independent on Sunday*, 9.

Commission for Racial Equality (1989a), *The Race Relations Act 1976: A guide for accommodation bureaux, landladies and landlords*, London: CRE.

Commission for Racial Equality (1989b), *The Race Relations Act 1976: A guide for estate agents and vendors*, London: CRE.

Consensus Development Conference (1986), 'Consensus Development Conference: treatment of primary breast cancer', *British Medical Journal*, 293: 946–7.

Cook, J. and Watt, S. (1989), 'Another expectation unfulfilled: black women and social services departments', in C. Hallett (ed.), *Women and Social Services Departments*, Hemel Hempstead: Harvester Wheatsheaf.

Cook, J. and Watt, S. (1992), 'Racism, women and poverty', in C. Glendinning and J. Millar (eds), *Women and Poverty in Britain in the 1990s*, Hemel Hempstead: Harvester Wheatsheaf.

Cook, J. and Watt, S. (1993), 'Racism: whose liberation? Implications for women's studies', in J. Aaron and S. Walby (eds), *Out of the Margins: Women's studies in the nineties*, London: Falmer Press.

Cooper, W. (1979), *No Change*, London: Arrow.

Corob, A. (1987), *Working with Depressed Women*, Aldershot: Gower.

Cousins, C. (1987), *Controlling Social Welfare*, Hemel Hempstead: Harvester Wheatsheaf.

Dale, J. and Foster, P. (1986), *Feminists and State Welfare*, London: Routledge & Kegan Paul.

Dalley, G. (1988), *Ideologies of Caring: Rethinking community and collectivism*, Macmillan Women in Society Series, London: Macmillan.

Darke, J. (1987), 'Report from housing workshop', *Planning and Housing Policies: Their effect on women*, Sheffield: Sheffield Centre for Environmental Research.

Darke, J. (1989), 'Problem without a name', *Roof* (March/April): 31.

Darke, J. (1994), 'Women and the meaning of home', in R. Gilroy and R. Woods (eds), *Housing Women*, London and New York: Routledge.

Darley, J. (1993), 'A background to recent UK education reforms and their possible gender implications', paper presented to the British Educational Research Association, Liverpool University.

David, M. (1993), *Parents, Gender and Education Reform*, Cambridge: Polity Press.

Davies, B. and Ward, S. (1992), *Women and Personal Pensions*, EOC Research Series, London: HMSO.

Davies, C. and Rosser, J. (1986), *Processes of Discrimination: A report on a study of women working in the NHS*, London: DHSS.

Davies, H. and Joshi, H. (1994), 'Sex, sharing and the distribution of income', *Journal of Social Policy*, 23, 3: 30–40.

Davis, A. (1982), *Sex, Race and Class*, London: Women's Press.

Davis, A. (1991), 'Hazardous lives: social work in the 1980s. A view from the left', in M. Loney, R. Bocock, J. Clarke, A. Cochrane, G. Peggotty and M. Wilson (eds), *The State or the Market: Politics and welfare in contemporary Britain*, London: Sage.

Dean, H. and Taylor-Gooby, P. (1990), 'Inequality and occupational sick pay', *Policy and Politics*, 18, 2: 145–50.

Dean, H. and Taylor-Gooby, P. (1992), *Dependency Culture: The explosion of a myth*, Hemel Hempstead: Harvester Wheatsheaf.

Dearing, R. (1994), Review of the National Curriculum and its Assessment, London: Schools Curriculum and Assessment Authority.

Deem, R. (1978), *Women and Schooling*, London: Routledge.

Deem, R. (1990), 'Governing by gender? School governing bodies after the Education Reform Act', in P. Abbott and C. Wallace (eds), *Gender, Power and Sexuality*, London: Macmillan.

Deem, R. (1994a), 'Free marketeers or good citizens? Education policy and lay participation in the administration of schools', *British Journal of Educational Studies*, 42, 1: 23–37.

Deem, R. (1994b), 'The school, the parent, the banker and the politician: what can we learn from the English experience of involving lay people in the site based management of schools?', paper delivered at the American Educational Research Association Annual Meeting, New Orleans.

Deem, R. (1994c), 'The organisational practices of school government: modernist or postmodernist?', paper presented to the CEDAR International Conference, Changing Educational Structures: Policy and Practice, University of Warwick.

Deem, R. and Brehony, K. (1993), 'Reforming school governing bodies: a sociological investigation', end-of-project report to the Economic and Social Research Council, Swindon.

Deem, R., Brehony, K. J. and Heath, S. (1995), *Active Citizenship and the Governing of Schools*, Buckingham: Open University Press.

Dekker Committee (Commissie Structuur en Financiering Gezondheidszorg) (1987), *Willingness to Change* (Bereidheid tot verandering), The Hague: DOP.

Delphy, C. (1984), *Close to Home: A materialist analysis of women's oppression*, London: Hutchinson.

Department of the Environment (DoE) (1993), *Housing in England: Housing trailers to the 1988 and 1991 Labour Force Surveys*, London: HMSO.

Department of the Environment, Scottish Development Department and Welsh Office (1992), *Housing and Construction Statistics 1981–1991, Gt Britain*, London, HMSO.

Department of Health (DoH), (1993), *Employers and Carers*, London: HMSO.

Department of Health (1994a), *A Wider Strategy for Research and Development Relating to Personal Social Services*, report to the Director of Research and Development, Department of Health by an Independent Review Group, London: HMSO.

Department of Health (1994b), *Implementing Caring for People: Care management*, London: Department of Health.

Department of Health and Social Security (DHSS) (1981a), *Growing Older*, Cmnd 8173, London: HMSO.

Department of Health and Social Security (1981b), *Care in Action: A handbook of policies and priorities for the health and personal social services in England*, London: HMSO.

Department of Health and Social Security (1987), *Health and Personal Social Services for England*, London: HMSO.

Department of Social Security (DSS) (1993), *Social Security Statistics 1993*, London: HMSO.

Department of Social Security (1994), *Households below Average Income 1979–1991/92*, London: HMSO.

Dex, S. (1985), *The Sexual Division of Work*, Hemel Hempstead: Harvester Wheatsheaf.

Dex, S. (1987), *Women's Occupational Mobility: A lifetime perspective*, London: Macmillan.

Di Stefano, C. (1990), 'Dilemmas of difference: feminism, modernity and postmodernism', in L. Nicholson (ed.), *Feminism/Postmodernism*, New York and London: Routledge.

Dibblin, J. (1988), 'Jenny lives with Eric and Martin', *Roof* (November/December): 25–7.

Dilnot, A., Kay, J. and Morris, C. (1984), *The Reform of Social Security*, Oxford: Clarendon Press.

Dimnik, S.B. (1987), 'Stepfathers "at risk"? A study of father-substitutes on the child abuse registers in York', MSW thesis, University of York.

Dobash, R. and Dobash, R. (1992), *Women, Violence and Social Change*, London: Routledge.

Dominelli, L. (1986), *Anti-Racist Social Work*, London: Macmillan.

Dominelli, L. and McLeod, E. (1989), *Feminist Social Work*, London: Macmillan.

Donald, J. and Rattansi, A. (eds) (1992), *'Race', Culture and Difference*, London: Sage/Open University.

Doogan, K. (1993), *Labour Mobility and the Housing Market: The employer's response*, Bristol: SAUS.

Douglas, G., Hebenton, B. and Thomas, T. (1992), 'The right to found a family', *New Law Journal*, 142, 6547: 488–90.

Duncan, A., Giles, C. and Webb, S. (1994), *Social Security Reform and Women's Independent Income*, Manchester: Equal Opportunities Commission.

Edwards, R. (1993), *Mature Women Students*, London: Taylor & Francis.

Egerton, J. (1990), 'Out but not down: lesbian's experience of housing', *Feminist Review*, 36 (Autumn): 75–88.

Employment Department (1992a) *New Training Survey*, London: HMSO.

Employment Department (1992b), 'Women and the labour market: results from the 1991 Labour Force Survey', *Employment Gazette* (September): 433–59.

Employment Department (1993a), 'Labour force projections 1993–2006', *Employment Gazette* (April): 139–47.

Employment Department (1993b), 'Ethnic origins and the labour market', *Employment Gazette* (February): 25–43.

Employment Department (1993c), *New Earnings Survey 1993, Part A*, London: HMSO.

Employment Department (1994), *Labour Market Statistics: Summary statistics*, Press Notice, 15 June.

Employment Department/Kids Club Network (n.d.), *Taking the Initiative on Out of School Childcare: A guide to TECs*, London: HMSO.

Equal Opportunities Commission (EOC) (1988), *Women and Men in Britain: A research profile*, London: HMSO.

Equal Opportunities Commission (1993), *Formal Investigation into the Publicity Funded Vocational Training System in England and Wales*, Manchester: EOC.

Esam, P. and Berthoud, R. (1991), *Independent Benefits for Men and Women*, London: Policy Studies Institute.

Esping-Andersen, G (1990), *The Three Worlds of Welfare Capitalism*, London: Polity Press.

Ettore, E. (1992), *Woman and Substance Use*, Basingstoke: Macmillan.

Evans, D., Fentiman, I., McPherson, K., Asbury, D., Ponder, B. and Howell, A. (1994), 'Familial breast cancer', *British Medical Journal*, 308: 183–7.

Evason, E. (1991), 'Women and poverty', in C. Davies and E. McLaughlin (eds), *Women, Employment and Social Policy in Ireland: A problem postponed?*, Belfast: Policy Research Institute.

Evers, A. and Svetlik, I. (eds) (1993), *Balancing Pluralism: New welfare mixes in care for the elderly*, Aldershot: Avebury.

Evers, A. and van der Zanden, G. (eds) (1993), *Better Care for Dependent People Living at Home: Meeting the new agenda in services for the elderly*, Bunnik: Netherlands Institute of Gerontology.

Evetts, J. (1990), *Women in Primary Teaching*, London: Unwin Hyman.

Fanon, F. (1986), *Black Skin, White Masks*, with a foreword by H. Bhaba, London: Pluto Press.

Faulder, C. (1993), 'The nation with the highest death rate debates prevention', *Women's Health Newsletter*, 19: 12–13.

Featherstone, M. and Hepworth, M. (1989), 'Ageing old age', in B. Bytheway, T. Keil, P. Allatt and A. Bryman (eds), *Becoming and Being Old*, London: Sage.

Featherstone, M. and Hepworth, M. (1990), 'Images of ageing', in J. Bond and P. Coleman (eds), *Ageing in Society: An introduction to social gerontology*, London: Sage.

Ferris, J. (1991), 'Green politics and the future of welfare', in N. Manning (ed.), *Social Policy Review 1990–1991*, Harlow: Longman.

Finch, J. (1984), 'Community care: developing non-sexist alternatives', *Critical Social Policy*, 9: 6–18.

Finch, J. (1989), *Family Obligations and Social Change*, Oxford: Polity Press.

Finch, J. (1990), 'The politics of community care in Britain', in C. Ungerson (ed.), *Gender and Caring*, Hemel Hempstead: Harvester Wheatsheaf.

Finch, J. and Groves, D. (1980), 'Community care and the family: a case for equal opportunities?', *Journal of Social Policy*, 9, 4: 487–511.

Finch, J. and Groves, D. (eds) (1983), *A Labour of Love: Women, work and caring*, London: Routledge & Kegan Paul.

Finch, J. and Mason, J. (1990), 'Filial obligations and kin support for elderly people', *Ageing and Society*, 10: 151–76.

Finch, J. and Mason, J. (1993), *Negotiating Family Responsibilities*, London: Routledge.

Firestone, S. (1974), *The Dialectic of Sex: The case for feminist revolution*, New York: Morrow.

Fitzhugh, A. (1993), *The Fitzhugh Directory of Independent Health Care Financial Information 1993–1994*, London: Health Care Information Services.

Flintoff, A. (1993), 'Gender, physical education and initial teacher education', in J. Evans (ed.), *Equality, Education and Physical Education*, London: Falmer Press.

Fowler, N. (1984), 'The enabling role of Social Services Departments', speech to the Joint Social Services Annual Conference, Buxton, 27 September.

Fowler, N. (1986), Speech to the Joint Social Services Annual Conference, Cardiff, 19 September, on the theme of Community Care.

Fraser, N. (1989), *Unruly Practices: Power, discourse and gender in contemporary social theory*, Cambridge: Polity Press.

Fraser, N. and Nicholson, L. (1990), 'Social criticism without philosophy: an encounter between feminism and postmodernism', in L. Nicholson (ed.), *Feminism/Postmodernism*, New York and London: Routledge.

Friedman, M. (1962), *Capitalism and Freedom*, Chicago: Chicago University Press.

Fugh-Berman, A. and Epstein, S. (1992), 'Tamoxifen: disease prevention or disease substitution?', *The Lancet*, 340: 1143–4.

Furstenburg, F. and Cherlin, A.J. (1991), *Divided Families: What happens to children when parents part*, Cambridge, Mass.: Harvard University Press.

Gangar, K. and Key, E. (1991), 'Presentation of menopausal symptoms', *Well Woman Team*, 4: 8–9.

186 References

George, M. (1994), 'Racism in nursing', *Nursing Standard*, 8, 18: 20–1.

George, V. and Wilding, P. (1994), *Welfare and Ideology*, Hemel Hempstead: Harvester Wheatsheaf.

Giddens, A. (1984), *The Constitution of Society: Outline of the theory of structuration*, Cambridge: Polity Press.

Gilman, S.L. (1992), 'Black bodies, white bodies: toward an iconography of female sexuality in late nineteenth-century art, medicine and literature', in J. Donald and A. Rattansi (eds), *'Race', Culture and Difference*, London: Sage/Open University.

Gilroy, P. (1987), *There Ain't no Black in the Union Jack*, London: Hutchinson.

Gilroy, P. (1993), *The Black Atlantic: Modernity and double consciousness*, London: Verso.

Gilroy, R. (1993), *Good Practices in Equal Opportunities*, Aldershot: Avebury.

Gilroy, R. (1994) 'Women and owner occupation in Britain: first the prince, and then the palace?', in R. Gilroy and R. Woods (eds), *Housing Women*, London and New York: Routledge.

Ginn, J. (1993), 'Grey power: age-based organisations' response to structured inequalities', *Critical Social Policy*, 13, 2: 23–47.

Ginn, J. and Arber, S. (1993), 'Pension penalties: the gendered division of occupational welfare', *Work, Employment and Society*, 7, 1: 47–70.

Ginn, J. and Arber, S. (1994), 'Heading for hardship: how the British pension system has failed women', in S. Baldwin and J. Falkingham (eds), *Social Security and Social Change*, Hemel Hempstead: Harvester Wheatsheaf.

Ginsburg, M., Cooper, S., *et al.*, (1990), 'National and world system explanations of educational reform', *Comparative Education Review*, 34, 4: 474–99.

Gipps, C. and Murphy, P. (1994), *A Fair Test*, Milton Keynes: Open University Press.

Gledhill, A. *et al.* (1989), *Who Cares? Children at risk and social services*, Policy Studies no. 111, London: Centre for Policy Studies.

Glendinning, C. (1992), *The Costs of Informal Care: Looking inside the household*, London: HMSO.

Glendinning, C. and Millar, J. (1987), *Women and Poverty in Britain*, Hemel Hempstead: Harvester Wheatsheaf.

Glendinning, C. and Millar, J. (eds) (1992), *Women and Poverty in Britain* (2nd edition), Hemel Hempstead: Harvester Wheatsheaf.

Glendinning, C. and Millar, J. (1994), 'Women and welfare: still on the margins', *Poverty* (Summer): 6–8.

Glennerster, H. (1992), *Paying for Welfare: The 1990s*, Hemel Hempstead: Harvester Wheatsheaf.

Glennerster, H. and Midgley, J. (eds) (1991), *The Radical Right and the Welfare State: An international assessment*, Hemel Hempstead: Harvester Wheatsheaf.

Glithero, A. (1986), 'Lending to women: dispelling the myths', *Housing Review*, 35, 6: 202–3.

Goffman, E. (1961), *Asylums: Essays on the social situation of mental patients and other inmates*, Harmondsworth: Penguin.

Goldner, V., Penn, P., Sheinberg, M. and Walker, G. (1990), 'Love and violence: gender paradoxes in volatile attachments', *Family Process*, 29, 4: 343–64.

Goodman, A. and Webb, S. (1994), *For Richer, for Poorer: The changing distribution of income in the UK, 1961–1991*, London: Institute for Fiscal Studies.

Gordon, L. (1989), *Heroes of their Own Lives: The politics and history of family violence*, London: Virago.

Gordon, P. (1986), 'Racism and social security', *Critical Social Policy*, 17: 23–40.

Gordon, P. (1989), *Citizenship for Some? Race and government policy 1979–1989*, London: Runnymede Trust.

Gordon, P. and Newnham, A. (1985), *Passport to Benefits? Racism in social security*, London: Child Poverty Action Group.

Goss, S. and Brown, H. (1991), *Equal Opportunities for Women in the NHS*, London: NHS Management Executive.

Gough, I. (1979), *The Political Economy of the Welfare State*, London: Macmillan.

Government Statistical Services (1993), *Education Statistics for the UK 1992*, London: HMSO.

Graham, H. (1983), 'Caring: a labour of love', in J. Finch and D. Groves (eds), *A Labour of Love: Women, work and caring*, London: Routledge & Kegan Paul.

Graham, H. (1987), 'Being poor: perceptions and coping strategies of lone mothers', in J. Brannen and G. Wilson (eds), *Give and Take in Families*, London: Allen & Unwin.

Graham, H. (1991), 'The concept of caring in feminist research: the case of domestic service', *Sociology*, 25, 1: 61–78.

Graham, H. (1993a), 'Feminist perspectives on caring', in J. Bornat, C. Pereira, D. Pilgrim and F. Williams (eds), *Community Care: A reader*, Basingstoke: Macmillan.

Graham, H. (1993b), *When Life's a Drag: Women, smoking and disadvantage*, London: HMSO.

Green, H. (1988), *Informal Carers*, OPCS Series, GHS, Supplement A, London: HMSO.

Green, K. (1993), 'Returning to the primary classroom', *Journal of Teacher Development*, 2, 3: 134–40.

Griffiths Report (1988), *Community Care: Agenda for action*, London: HMSO.

Grimsley, M. and Bhat, A. (1988), 'Health', in A. Bhat, R. Carr-Hill and S. Ohris (eds), *Britain's Black Population: A new perspective*, The Radical Statistics Race Group, Aldershot: Gower.

Groves, D. (1992), 'Occupational pension provision and women's poverty in old age', in C. Glendinning and J. Millar (eds), *Women and Poverty: The 1990s*, Hemel Hempstead: Harvester Wheatsheaf.

Gunew, S. (1992), *Feminism: Critique and construct*, London: Routledge.

Gurnah, A. (1989) 'Translating equality policies into practice', *Critical Social Policy*, 27: 110–24.

Hackett, G. and Pyke, N. (1994), 'Secrets of the quango tango', *Times Educational Supplement*, 22 April, 13–14.

Hakim, C. (1979), *Occupational Segregation*, Research Paper no. 44, London: Employment Department.

Hakim, C. (1993), 'The myth of rising female employment work', *Employment and Society*, 7, 1: 97–120.

Hall, S. (1978), 'Racism and reaction', in *Five Views of Multi-racial Britain*, London: Commission for Racial Equality.

Hallett, C. (1982), *The Personal Social Services in Local Government*, London: Allen & Unwin.

Hallett, C. (ed.) (1989), *Women and Social Services Departments*, Hemel Hempstead: Harvester Wheatsheaf.

Halpin, D. and Troyna, B. (1994), 'Lessons in school reform from Great Britain? The politics of education policy borrowing', paper presented to the American Educational Research Association, New Orleans.

Ham, C. and Hill, M. (1984), *The Policy Process in the Modern Capitalist State*, Hemel Hempstead: Harvester Wheatsheaf.

Hanmer, J. and Stratham, D. (1988), *Women and Social Work: Towards a woman centred practice*, London: Macmillan.

Harding, S. (ed.) (1987), *Feminism and Methodology: Social science issues*, Milton Keynes: Open University.

Harding, T. (ed.) (1992), *Who Owns Welfare? Questions on the social services agenda*, Social Services Policy Forum, paper no. 2, London: NISW.

Harris, S. (1994), 'School inspection and equal opportunities', paper presented to the CEDAR International Conference, Changing Educational Structures: Policy and Practice, University of Warwick.

Hart, J. and Richardson, D. (1981), *The Theory and Practice of Homosexuality*, London: Routledge & Kegan Paul.

Hatchett, W. (1990), 'Private care homes boom or bust?', *Community Care*, 26 July.

Hayden, J. (1991), 'Women in general practice', *British Medical Journal*, 303: 733–4.

Health Education Authority (HEA) (1991), *Pregnancy Book*, London: HEA.

Heery, E. and Kelly, J. (1994), 'Professional, participative and managerial unionism: an interpretation of change in trade unions', *Work, Employment and Society*, 8, 1: 1–22.

Hennings, J. (1993), *Asian Women's Experience of Maternity Care*, Department of Social Policy and Social Work, University of Manchester.

Henwood, M. (1992), 'Demographic and family change', in T. Harding (ed.), *Who Owns Welfare? Questions on the social services agenda*, Social Services Policy Forum, paper no. 2, London: NISW.

Her Majesty's Stationery Office (HMSO) (1989), *Caring for People*, Cmnd 849, London: HMSO.

Herman, J. and Hirschman, L. (1981), *Father–Daughter Incest*, Cambridge, Mass.: Harvard University Press.

Hernes, H. (1987), 'Women and the welfare state: the transition from private to public dependence', in A. Showstack Sassoon (ed.), *Women and the State*, London: Hutchinson.

Hester, M. and Pearson, C. (1993), 'Domestic violence, mediation and child contact arrangements: issues from current research', *Family Mediation*, 3, 2: 3–6.

Hester, M. and Radford, L. (1992), 'Domestic violence and access arrangements for children in Denmark and Britain', *Journal of Social Welfare and Family Law*, 1: 57–70.

Higgins, J. (1988), *The Business of Medicine Private Health Care in Britain*, London: Macmillan.

Higgins, J. (1989), 'Defining community care: realities and myths', *Social Policy and Administration*, 23, 1: 3–15.

Hill, M. (1993), *An Introduction to Social Policy* (4th edition), Oxford: Blackwell.

Hill Collins, P. (1990), *Black Feminist Thought*, London: Routledge.

Hills, J. (ed.) (1990), *The State of Welfare*, Oxford: Clarendon Press.

Hindess, B. (1987), *Freedom, Equality and the Market*, London: Tavistock.

Hirsh, W., Hayday, S., Yeates, J. and Callender, C. (1992), *Beyond the Career Break: A study of professional and managerial women returning to work after having a child*, Brighton: Institute of Manpower Studies.

Hockey, J. and James, A. (1993), *Growing up and Growing Old: Ageing and dependency in the lifecourse*, London: Sage.

Hoff, L. (1990), *Battered Women as Survivors*, London: Routledge.

Holland, J., Ramazanoglu, C., Sharpe, S. and Thomson, R. (1992), 'Pressured pleasure: young women and the negotiation of sexual boundaries', *Sociological Review*, 40, 4: 645–74.

Holly, L. (1989), 'My Nan said, "Sure you're not pregnant?": school girl mothers', in L. Holly (ed.), *Girls and Sexuality*, Milton Keynes: Open University Press.

Holterman, S. and Clarke, K. (1992), 'Parents, employment rights and childcare', Research Discussion Series no. 4, Manchester: Equal Opportunities Commission.

hooks, b. (1981), *Ain't I a Woman? Black women and feminism*, Boston, Mass.: South End Press.
hooks, b. (1984), *Feminist Theory: From margin to center*, Boston, Mass.: South End Press.
hooks, b. (1990), *Yearning: Race, gender and cultural politics*, Boston, Mass.: South End Press.
Hooper, C.A. (1992), *Mothers Surviving Child Sexual Abuse*, London: Routledge.
Hooper, C.A. (1994), 'Do families need fathers? The impact of divorce on children', in A. Mullender and B. Morley (eds), *Children Living with Domestic Violence*, London: Whiting & Birch.
House of Commons (1985), *Community Care: Second report from the Social Services Committee*, Session 1984–85, vol. 1, London: HMSO.
Howarth, K. (1991), 'Are ante natal tests unhealthy?', *GP*, 3 May, 56–7.
Hughes, M. and Hunter, T. (1993), 'Why the personal pension storm is gathering force', *The Guardian*, 11 December.
Hull, G., Bell Scott, P. and Smith, B. (eds) (1981), *All the Women are White, All the Blacks are Men, but Some of us are Brave: Black women's studies*, New York: Feminist Press.
Humm, M. (ed.) (1993), *Feminisms: A reader*, Hemel Hempstead: Harvester Wheatsheaf.
Income Data Services (IDS) (1991a), *Sick Pay Schemes*, Study 475, London: IDS.
Income Data Services (1991b), *Maternity Leave and Career Breaks*, Study 476, London: IDS.
Income Data Services (1993), *Private Medical Insurance*, Study 527, London: IDS.
Incomes Data Services (1994), *Maternity Leave*, Study 550, London: IDS.
Institute of Housing (Women in Housing Working Party) (1987), *Relationship Breakdown*, London: Institute of Housing.
Jackson, S. (1995), 'Gender and homosexuality: a materialist, feminist analysis', in M. Maynard and J. Purvis (eds), *(Hetero)Sexual Politics*, London: Taylor & Francis.
Jaffe, P.G., Wolfe, D. A. and Wilson, S.K. (1990), *Children of Battered Women*, London: Sage.
Jaggar, A. (1983), *Feminist Politics and Human Nature*, Hemel Hempstead: Harvester Wheatsheaf.
James, M. and Busia, A.P.A. (eds) (1993), *Theorizing Black Feminisms: The visionary pragmatism of black women*, New York: Routledge.
Jamieson, A. (1989), 'A new age for older people? Policy shifts in health and social care', *Social Science and Medicine*, 29, 3: 445 54.
Jamieson, A. (ed.) (1991), *Home Care for Older People in Europe: A comparison of policies and practices*, Oxford: Oxford University Press.
Jani-Le Bris, H. (1993), *Family Care of Dependent Older People in the European Community*, Luxembourg: Office for Official Publications of the European Communities.
Jarman, R. (1994), 'Legislated learning: aspects of Northern Ireland experience', *Journal of Teacher Development*, 3, 3.
Jeffcoate, N. (1957), *Principles of Gynaecology*, London: Butterworth.
Jenkins, S.P. (1991), 'Poverty measurement and the within household distribution', *Journal of Social Policy*, 20, 4: 457–83.
Jenkins, S.P. (1994), *Winners and Losers: A portrait of the UK income distribution during the 1990s*, University of Swansea: Department of Economics.
Johansson, L. (1993), 'Swedes test new strategies', *Ageing International*, 20, 2: 42–5.
Johnson, N. (1987), *The Welfare State in Transition*, Hemel Hempstead: Harvester Wheatsheaf.
Johnson, N. (1990), *Reconstructing the Welfare State: A decade of change 1980–1990*, London: Harvester Wheatsheaf.
Johnson-Reagan, B. (1983) 'Coalition politics; turning the century', in Smith, B., *Home Girls: A black feminist anthology*, New York: Kitchen Table: Women of Colour Press.
Jones, T. (1993), *Britain's Ethnic Minorities*, London: Policy Studies Institute.

Joshi, H. and Davies, H. (1991), 'Pension splitting and divorce', *Fiscal Studies*, 12, 4: 69–71.

Joshi, H. and Davies, H. (1991a), *The Pension Consequences of Divorce*, London: Centre for Economic Policy Research.

Joshi, H. and Davies, H. (1993), *Mothers' Human Capital and Child Care in Britain*, London: National Institute of Economic and Social Research.

Kane, P. (1991), *Women's Health: From womb to tomb*, London: Macmillan.

Keat, R. and Abercrombie, N. (1991), *Enterprise Culture*, London: Routledge.

Kelly, E. (1986), 'What makes women feel safe?', *Housing Review*, 35, 6: 198–200.

Kelly, L. (1988), 'How women define their experiences of violence', in K. Yllo and M. Bograd (eds), *Feminist Perspectives on Wife Abuse*, London: Sage.

Kelly, L. and Radford, J. (1990/1), 'Nothing really happened: the invalidation of women's experience of sexual violence', *Critical Social Policy*, 30: 39–53.

Kempson, E., Bryson, A. and Rowlingson, K. (1994), *Hard times? How poor families make ends meet*, London: Policy Studies Institute.

Keys, W. and Fernandes, C. (1990), *A Survey of School Governing Bodies*, Slough: National Foundation for Educational Research.

King's Fund (1990), *Racial Equality: The nursing profession*, Occasional Paper no. 6, London: King's Fund.

Kirkwood, C. (1993), *Leaving Abusive Partners*, London: Sage.

Klein, R. (1989), 'Doing it ourselves: self insemination', in R. Arditti, R. Klein, and S. Minden (eds), *Test Tube Women*, London: Pandora Press.

Klemi, P.J., Joensuu, H., Toikkanen, S., Tuominen, J., Räsänen, O., Trykkö, J. and Parvinen, I. (1992), 'Aggressiveness of breast cancers found with and without screening', *British Medical Journal*, 304: 467–9.

Knowles, C. and Mercer, S. (1992), 'Feminism and anti-racism: an exploration of political possibilities', in J. Donald and A. Rattansi (eds), *'Race', Culture and Difference*, London: Sage/Open University.

Knupfer, G. (1991) 'Abstaining for foetal health: the fiction that even light drinking is dangerous', *British Journal of Addiction*, 86: 1063–73.

Kraan, R., Baldock, J., Davies, B., Evers, A., Johansson, L., Knapen, M., Thorslund, M. and Tunissen, C. (1991) *Care for the Elderly: Significant innovations in three European countries*, Frankfurt-on-Main: Campus Verlag.

LACSAB/ADSS (1990), *Social Services Employment Survey 1989*, London: Local Authorities Conditions of Service Advisory Board.

Ladner, J. (1971), *Tomorrow's Tomorrow: The black woman*, New York: Doubleday.

Laing, W. (1990), *Care of Elderly People Market Survey 1990/91*, London: Laing & Buisson.

Laing, W. (1991), *Private Health Care Insurance and the Future of Private Health Care in the UK*, Special Market Report, London: Laing & Buisson.

Laing, W. (1992), *Laing's Review of Private Health Care 1992*, London: Laing & Buisson.

Laing, W. (1993a), *Financing Long-term Care: The crucial debate*, London: Age Concern England.

Laing, W. (1993b), *Laing's Review of Private Health Care 1993*, London: Laing & Buisson.

Land, H. (1983a), 'Poverty and gender: the distribution of resources within families', in M. Brown (ed.), *The Structure of Disadvantage*, London, Heinemann.

Land, H. (1983b), 'Who still cares for the family?', in J. Lewis (ed.), *Women, Welfare and Women's Rights*, London: Croom Helm.

Land, H. (1989), 'Who cares for the family?', *Journal of Social Policy*, 7, 3: 357–84.

Land, H. (1994), 'The demise of the male breadwinner – in practice but not in theory: a challenge for social security systems', in S. Baldwin and J. Falkingham (eds), *Social Security and Social Change: New challenges to the Beveridge Model*, Hemel Hempstead: Harvester Wheatsheaf.

Land, H. and Rose, H. (1985), 'Compulsory altruism for some or an altruistic society for all?', in P. Bean, J. Ferris and D. Whynes (eds), *In Defence of Welfare*, London: Tavistock.

Langan, M. and Clarke, J. (1994), 'Managing in the mixed economy of care', in J. Clarke, A. Cochrane and E. McLaughlin (eds), *Managing Social Policy*, London: Sage.

Langan, M. and Day, L. (eds) (1992), *Women, Oppression and Social Work Issues in Anti-Discriminatory Practice*, London: Routledge.

Larbie, J. (1985), *Black Women and the Maternity Services*, London: Training in Health and Race.

Law Commission (1990), *Family Law: The ground for divorce*, London: HMSO.

Law, W. (1992), 'Long time no see', *Human Resources* (Autumn): 131–4.

Lawrence, E. (1982), 'In the abundance of water the fool is thirsty: sociology and black "pathology" ', in Centre for Contemporary Political Studies (CSS), *The Empire Strikes Back*, London: Hutchinson.

Le Grand, J. (1982), *The Strategy of Equality*, London: Allen & Unwin.

Le Grand, J. and Bartlett, W. (eds) (1993), *Quasi-markets and Social Policy*, London: Macmillan.

Leat, D. (1992), 'Innovations and special schemes', in J. Twigg (ed.), *Carers: Research and practice*, London, HMSO.

Leila, H. and Elliott, P. (1987), *Infertility and In Vitro Fertilisation*, London: BMA.

Levin, E., Sinclair, I. and Gorbach, P. (1989), *Families, Services and Confusion in Old Age*, Aldershot: Gower.

Lewis, J. and Meredith, B. (1988), *Daughters who Care: Daughters caring for mothers at home*, London: Routledge.

Lister, R. (1992), *Women's Economic Dependency and Social Security*, Manchester: Equal Opportunities Commission.

Lister, R. (1994), ' "She has other duties": women, citizenship and social security', in S. Baldwin and J. Falkingham (eds), *Social Security and Social Change: New Challenges to the Beveridge Model*, Hemel Hempstead: Harvester Wheatsheaf.

Little, J., Peake, L. and Richardson, P. (1988) *Women in Cities*, London: Macmillan.

Logan, F. (1986), *Homelessness and Relationship Breakdown; How the law and housing policy affects women*, London: National Council for One Parent Families; London: Croom Helm.

Lonsdale, S. (1992), 'Patterns of paid work', in C. Glendinning and J. Millar (eds), *Women and Poverty in Britain: The 1990s*, Hemel Hempstead: Harvester Wheatsheaf.

Lord Chancellor's Department (1993), *Looking to the Future*, London: HMSO.

Lorde, A. (1984), 'An open letter to Mary Daly', in *Sister Outsider*, New York: Crossing Press.

Machin, S. and Waldfogel, J. (1994), *The Decline of the Male Breadwinner: Changing shares of husbands and wives' earnings in family income*, Welfare State Programme WSP/103, London: London School of Economics.

Macintyre, S. (1977), 'Old age as a social problem', in R. Dingwall *et al.* (eds), *Health Care and Health Knowledge*, London: Croom Helm.

Maclean, M. and Groves, D. (eds) (1991), *Women's Issues in Social Policy*, London: Routledge.

MacLennan, E. (1980), *Minimum Wages for Women*, Manchester: Equal Opportunities Commission/Low Pay Unit.

Maddock, S. and Parkin, D. (1994), 'Barriers to women doctors in the North Western Region', unpublished report for North West Regional Health Authority.

Madood, T. (1988), ' "Black" racial equality and Asian identity', *New Community*, 14, 3: 397–404.

Mama, A. (1984), 'Black women, the economic crisis and the British state', *Feminist Review*, 17: 21–36.

Mama, A. (1989), *The Hidden Struggle: Statutory and voluntary sector responses to violence against black women in the home*, London: London Race and Housing Research Unit.

Mama, A. (1993a), 'Problems with feminist analyses of the state', *Feminist Review*.

Mama, A. (1993b), 'Violence against black women: gender, race and state responses', in J. Walmsley, J. Reynolds, P. Shakespeare and R. Woolfe (eds), *Health, Welfare and Practice: Reflecting on roles and relationships*, London: Sage.

Marsh, A. and McKay, S. (1993a), 'Families, work and the use of childcare', *Employment Gazette* (August): 361–70.

Marsh, A. and McKay, S. (1993b), *Families, Work and Benefits*, London: Policy Studies Institute.

Marsh, A. and McKay, S. (1994), *Poor Smokers*, London: Policy Studies Institute.

Marshall, A. (1994), 'Orgasmic slavery: images of black female sexualities and the impact upon identity', paper presented at the forty-third Annual Conference of the British Sociological Association, held at the University of Central Lancashire, Preston, 28–31 March.

Marshall, B. (1994), *Engendering Modernity*, Cambridge: Polity Press.

Maternity Alliance (1985), *Multi-Racial Initiatives in Maternity Care*, London Maternity Alliance.

May, M. and Brunsdon, E. (1994), 'Workplace care in the mixed economy of welfare', in R. Page and J. Baldock (eds), *Social Policy Review 6*, Canterbury: Social Policy Association.

Maynard, M. (1985), 'The response of social workers to domestic violence', in J. Pahl (ed.), *Private Violence and Public Policy: The needs of battered women and the response of public services*, London: Routledge & Kegan Paul.

Mayo, M. and Weir, A. (1993), 'The future for feminist social policy?', in R. Page and J. Baldock (eds), *Social Policy Review 5*, Canterbury: Social Policy Association.

McCarthy, M. (1989), 'Personal social services', in M. McCarthy (ed.), *The New Politics of Welfare: An agenda for the 1990s*, London: Macmillan.

McCarthy, P. and Simpson, B. (1991), *Issues in Post Divorce Housing*. Aldershot: Avebury.

McDowell, L. (1983), 'Towards an understanding of the gender division of urban space', *Environment and Planning D: Society and Space*, 1: 59–72.

McIntosh, M. (1981), 'Feminism and social policy', *Critical Social Policy*, 1: 32–42.

McKay, S. and Marsh, A. (1994), *Lone Parents and Work*, Department of Social Security Research Report no. 25, London: HMSO.

McKeown, P. (1994), 'School governing bodies under local management of schools: the Northern Ireland experience', paper presented to the CEDAR Conference, University of Warwick.

McLaughlin, E. (1991), *Social Security and Community Care: The case of the Invalid Care Allowance*, London: HMSO.

McLaughlin, E. and Glendinning, C. (1994), 'Paying for care in Europe: is there a feminist approach?', in L. Hantrais and S. Mangen (eds), *Concepts and Contexts in International Comparisons: Family policy and the welfare of women*, Cross-National Research Papers, series 3, no. 3, University of Loughborough: Centre for European Studies.

McPherson, A. and Savage, W. (1987), 'Cervical cytology', in A. McPherson (ed.), *Women's Problems in General Practice*, Oxford: Oxford University Press.

McQuail, S. (1993), *No Childcare, No Training: TECSs, training providers and childcare allowances*, London: Daycare Trust/NCVO.

McRae, S. (1991), *Maternity Rights in Britain: The experience of women and employers*, London: Policy Studies Institute.

McRae, S. (1994), 'Labour supply after childbirth: do employers' policies make a difference?', *Sociology*, 28, 1: 99–122.

McTaggart, L. (1990), 'Screen violence', *What Doctors Don't Tell You*, 1, 6: 1–3.

McTaggart, L. (1993), 'Breast cancer: the unkindest cut', *What Doctors Don't Tell You*, 3, 11.

Meagre, N. and Court, G. (1993), *TECs and Equal Opportunities: A review paper*, Brighton: Institute of Manpower Studies.

Measor, L. (1989), 'Are you coming to see some dirty films today? Sex education and adolescent sexuality', in L. Holly (ed.), *Girls and Sexuality*, Milton Keynes: Open University Press.

Meredith, B. (1995), *The Community Care Handbook: The reformed system explained* (2nd edition), London: Age Concern England.

Middleton, S. (1993), 'A postmodern pedagogy for the sociology of women's education', in M. Arnot and K. Weiler (eds), *Feminism and Social Justice in Education*, London: Falmer Press.

Midwinter, E. (1986), *Caring for Cash: The issue of domiciliary private care*, London: Centre for Policy on Ageing.

Miles, A. (1988), *Women and Mental Illness*, Hemel Hempstead: Harvester Wheatsheaf.

Millar, J. (1987), 'Lone mothers', in C. Glendinning and J. Millar (eds), *Women and Poverty in Britain*, Hemel Hempstead: Harvester Wheatsheaf.

Millar, J. (1989), 'Social security, equality and women in the UK', *Policy and Politics*, 17, 4: 311–19.

Millar, J. (1994), 'Poor mothers and absent fathers', in H. Jones and J. Millar (eds), *The Politics of the Family*, Aldershot: Avebury.

Millar, J. (1996), 'Lone parents and social security policy in the UK', in S. Baldwin and J. Falkingham (eds), *Social Security and Social Change: New challenges to the Beveridge Model*, Hemel Hempstead: Harvester Wheatsheaf.

Millar, J. and Glendinning, C. (1987), 'Invisible women, invisible poverty', in C. Glendinning and J. Millar (eds), *Women and Poverty in Britain*, Hemel Hempstead: Harvester Wheatsheaf.

Millar, J. and Glendinning, C. (1989), 'Gender and poverty', *Journal of Social Policy*, 8, 3: 363–81.

Miller, M. (1990), *Bed and Breakfast: Women and homelessness today*, London: Women's Press.

Millett, K. (1970), *Sexual Politics*, London: Abacus; reprinted in 1977, London: Virago.

Milne, R. (1989), 'Tender topics for the NHS', *Health Service Journal* (5 January): 16–17.

Mishra, R. (1977), *Society and Social Policy*, London: Macmillan.

Mishra, R. (1984), *The Welfare State in Crisis*, Hemel Hempstead: Harvester Wheatsheaf.

Mohan, J. (1991), 'Privatisation in the British health sector', in J. Gabe, M. Calnan and M. Mury (eds), *The Sociology of the Health Service*, London: Routledge.

Mooney, J. (1993), *The Hidden Figure: Domestic violence in North London*, London Borough of Islington.

Mooney, J. and Young, J. (1993), 'Criminal deception', *New Statesman and Society*, 17/31 December.

Morley, B. (1993), 'Recent responses to "domestic violence" against women: a feminist critique', in R. Page and J. Baldock (eds), *Social Policy Review 5*, Canterbury: Social Policy Association.

Morris, J. (1991–2), ' "Us" and "them"? Feminist research, community care and disability', *Critical Social Policy*, 33: 22–39.

Morris, J. and Winn, M. (1990), *Housing and Social Inequality*, London: Hilary Shipman.

Muir, J. and Ross, M. (1993), *Housing the Poorer Sex*, London: London Housing Unit.

Munro, M. and Smith, S.J. (1989), 'Gender and housing: broadening the research debate', *Housing Studies*, 4, 1: 81–93.

Murray, I. (1994), 'Training the unemployed? Low level qualification and drop-out', *Unemployment Unit Working Brief*, 57 (August).

NACAB (1994), *Child Support: One year on. CAB evidence on the first year of the child support scheme*, London: NACAB.

Nanton, P. (1992), 'Official statistics and problems of inappropriate ethnic classification', *Policy and Politics*, 20, 4: 277–85.

NATFHE (1993), *Survey of Governing Bodies of FE Colleges*, London: NATFHE.

National Association of Health Authorities and Trusts (n.d.), *Where are the Good Women?*, London: NAHAT.

National Childbirth Trust (1991), Memorandum to the House of Commons Health Committee, *House of Commons (1990–91)*, 430 II.

National Steering Group on Equal Opportunities for Women (1987), 'Equal opportunities for women in the NHS', cited in S. Goss and H. Brown (1991), *Equal Opportunities for Women in the N.H.S.*, London, NHS Management Executive: Department of Health.

Nationwide Anglia Building Society (1989), *Lending to Women 1980–1988*, London: Nationwide Anglia Building Society.

Nationwide Anglia Building Society (1994), *House Prices in 1994: Fourth quarter*, London: Nationwide Anglia Building Society.

NCOPF (1994), *The Child Support Agency's First Year: The lone parent case*, London: NCOPF.

New Earnings Survey (1992), Department of Employment, London: HMSO.

Newman, J. (1994), The limits of management: gender and the politics of change', in J. Clarke, *et al.* (eds), *Managing Social Policy*, London: Sage.

Newnham, J.P., *et al.* (1993), 'Effects of frequent ultrasound during pregnancy: a randomised controlled trial', *The Lancet*, 342: 887–91.

Nicholl, J.P., Beeby, N.R. and Williams, B.T. (1989), *Comparison of Short Stay Independent Hospitals in England and Wales*, Sheffield: University of Sheffield.

Nicholson, L. (ed.) (1990), *Feminism/Postmodernism*, New York and London: Rouledge.

Nijkamp, P., Pacolet, J., Spinnewyn, H., Vollering, A., Wilderom, C. and Winters, S. (1991), *Services for the Elderly in Europe: A cross-national comparative study*, Leuven: Katholieke Universiteit.

Nissel, M., and Bonnerjea, L. (1982), *Family Care of the Handicapped Elderly: Who pays?*, London: Policy Studies Institute.

Norman, A. (1985), *Triple Jeopardy: Growing old in a second homeland*, London: Centre for Policy on Ageing.

Norris, P. (1986), *Politics and Sexual Equality*, Hemel Hempstead: Harvester Wheatsheaf.

O'Connor, J. (1973), *The Fiscal Crisis of the State*, New York: St Martin's Press.

Oakley, A. (1980), *Women Confined: Towards a sociology of childbirth*, Oxford: Martin Robinson.

Oakley, A. (1987), 'Home birth; a class privilege', *New Society*, 6 November, p. 27.

Office of Population Censuses and Surveys (OPCS) (1989), *The General Household Survey 1987*, London: HMSO.

Office of Population Censuses and Surveys (1991), *Marriage and Divorce Statistics*, Series FM2 no. 19, London: HMSO.

Office of Population Censuses and Surveys (1992), *General Household Survey*, London: HMSO.

Office of Population Censuses and Surveys (1993), *The General Household Survey 1991*, London: HMSO.

OHE (1987), *Women's Health Today*, London: OHE.

Oliver, M. (1990), *The Politics of Disablement*, Basingstoke: Macmillan.

Oppenheim, C. (1993), *Poverty the Facts*, London: Child Poverty Action Group.

Pahl, J. (1980), 'Patterns of money management within marriage', *Journal of Social Policy*, 9, 3: 313–35.

Pahl, J. (1989), *Money and Marriage*, London: Macmillan.

Parker, G. (1990), *With Due Care and Attention: A review of research on informal care* (2nd edition), London: Family Policy Studies Centre.

Parker, G. and Lawton, D. (1990), *Further Analysis of the 1985 General Household Survey Data on Informal Care. Report 2: The consequences of caring*, York: Social Policy Research Unit, University of York.

Parker, H. (1993), *Citizen's Income and Women*, BIRG Discussion Paper no. 2, London: Citizens' Income.

Parker, H. and Parker, S. (1986), 'Father–daughter sexual abuse: an emerging perspective', *American Journal of Orthopsychiatry*, 56, 4: 531–49.

Parmar, P. (1982), 'Gender, race and class: Asian women in resistance', in Centre for Contemporary Cultural Studies, *The Empire Strikes Back: Race and racism in 70s Britain*, London: Hutchinson.

Parmar, P. (1988), 'Gender, race and power', in P. Cohen and H.S. Bains (eds), *Multi-Racist Britain*, London: Macmillan.

Pascall, G. (1983), 'Women and social welfare', in P. Bean and S. Macpherson (eds), *Approaches to Welfare*, London: Routledge & Kegan Paul.

Pascall, G. (1986), *Social Policy: A feminist analysis*, London: Tavistock.

Pateman, C. (1988), *The Sexual Contract*, Cambridge: Polity Press.

Payne, S. (1991), *Women, Health and Poverty: An introduction*, Hemel Hempstead: Harvester Wheatsheaf.

Phillips, A. (1992), 'Feminism, equality and difference', in L. McDowell and R. Pringle (eds), *Defining Women: Social institutions and gender divisions*, Cambridge: Polity Press.

Phillips, J. (1992), *Private Residential Care: The admissions process and reactions of the public sector*, Aldershot: Avebury.

Phillipson, C. (1982), *Capitalism and the Construction of Old Age*, Basingstoke: Macmillan.

Phizacklea, A. (ed.) (1984), *One Way Ticket: Migration and female labour*, London: Routledge & Kegan Paul.

Phizacklea, A. (ed.) (1994), 'A single or segregated market: gendered and racialised divisions', in H. Afshar and M. Maynard (eds), *The Dynamics of 'Race' and Gender: Some feminist interventions*, London: Taylor & Francis.

Pierson, C. (1991), *Beyond the Welfare State*, Cambridge: Polity Press.

Piper, C. (1993), *The Responsible Parent: A study of divorce mediation*, Hemel Hempstead: Harvester Wheatsheaf.

Pollard, A., Broadfoot, P., *et al.* (1994), 'Changing English primary schools? A cautionary analysis', paper presented to the American Educational Research Association, New Orleans.

Pollock, S. (1984), 'Refusing to take women seriously: side effects; and the politics of contraception', in R. Arditti, R. Klein and S. Mindle (eds), *Test-Tube Women*, London: Pandora.

Popay, J. and Jones, G. (1990), 'Patterns of health and illness among lone parents', *Journal of Social Policy*, 19, 4: 499–535.

Prendergast, S. (1989), 'Girls' experience of menstruation in school', in L. Holly (ed.), *Girls and Sexuality*, Milton Keynes: Open University Press.

Prescott-Clarke, P., Clemens, S. and Park, A. (1994), *Routes into Local Authority Housing*, Department of the Environment, London: HMSO.

Propper, C. and Maynard, A. (1989), *The Market for Private Insurance in Britain*, York: Centre for Health Economics.

Qureshi, H. and Walker, A. (1989), *The Caring Relationship: Elderly people and their families*, Basingstoke: Macmillan.

Ramazanoglu, C. (1989), *Feminism and the Contradictions of Oppression*, London: Routledge.

Randhawa, K. (1986), 'Late booking: whose problem is it? *Maternity Action* (July/August): 9.

Rao, N. (1990), *Black Women in Public Housing*, London: Black Women in Housing Group.

Rattansi, A. (1992), 'Changing the subject? Racism, culture and education', in J. Donald and A. Rattansi (eds), *'Race', Culture and Difference*, London: Sage/Open University.

RCOG (1983), *Report of the RCOG Ethics Committee on In Vitro Fertilisation and Embryo Replacement or Transfer*, London: RCOG.

Reid, K. (1985), 'Choice of method', in N. London (ed.), *Handbook of Family Planning*, Edinburgh: Churchill Livingstone.

Rein, M. (1985), 'Women, employment and social welfare', in R. Klein and M. O'Higgins (eds), *The Future of Welfare*, Oxford: Blackwell.

Reynolds, K. (1993), 'Who pays the bills? Gender, race, class and local management', paper presented to the British Educational Research Association, Liverpool.

Rice, R. (1991), 'Law Society reports rise in number of women solicitors', *Financial Times*, 15 October.

Rich, A. (1980), 'Compulsory heterosexuality and lesbian existence', *Signs*, 5, 4: 631–60.

Richardson, J. (1993), 'The selection and recruitment of male and female head teachers', unpublished MA dissertation, Lancaster University.

Riddell, S. (1992), *Gender and the Politics of the Curriculum*, London: Routledge.

Riley, D. (1988), *Am I that Name? Feminism and the category of 'woman' in history*, London: Macmillan.

Ringen, S. (1988), 'Direct and indirect measures of poverty', *Journal of Social Policy*, 17, 3: 351–66.

Roberts, M. (1991), *Living in a Man-made World: Gender assumptions in modern housing design*, London and New York: Routledge.

Roberts, M., *et al.* (1990), 'Edinburgh trial of screening for breast cancer: mortality at seven years', *The Lancet*, 335: 241–6.

Robinson, J. (1981), 'Cervical cancer: a feminist critique', *Times Health Supplement*, 27 November.

Rodgers, A. (1991), Letter in *British Medical Journal*, 302: 1401.

Roll, J. (1992), *Understanding Poverty: A guide to the concepts and measures*, London: Family Policy Studies Centre.

Ross, S.K. (1989), 'Cervical cytology screening and government policy', *British Medical Journal*, 299: 101–4.

Rubery, J. and Fagan, C. (1993), *Occupational Segregation of Women and Men in the European Community*, Luxemburg: Social Europe Supplement 3/93, CEC.

Rubery, J. and Fagan, C. (1994), 'Occupational segregation: plus ça change . . . ?', in R. Lindley (ed.), *Labour Market Structures and Prospects for Women*, Manchester: Equal Opportunities Commission.

Rubin, G. (1975), 'The traffic in women', in R. Reiter (ed.), *Toward an Anthropology of Women*, New York: Monthly Review Press.

Russell, D. (1984), *Sexual Exploitation*, London: Sage.

Sainsbury, E. (1975), *The Personal Social Services*, London: Pitman.

Savage, W. (1991), Memorandum submitted to the House of Commons Health Committee, House of Commons (1991–2), 29 III.

Saville, J. (1957/8), 'The welfare state: an historical approach', *New Reasoner*, 3, 1: 5–25.

Schopflin, P. (1991), *Dépendance et solidarité: mieux aider les personnes âgées. Rapport de la Commission du Commissariat Général au Plan*, Paris: La Documentation Française.

Schorr, A. (1992), *The Personal Social Services: An outside view*, York: Joseph Rowntree Foundation.

Secretary of State for Health (1991), *The Health of the Nation*, Cm. 1523, London: HMSO.

Seebohm Report (1968), *Report of the Committee on Local Authority and Allied Personal Social Services*, Cmnd 3703, London: HMSO.

Segal, L. (1987), *Is the Future Female? Troubled thoughts on contemporary feminism*, London: Virago.

Seldon, A. (1957), *Pensions in a Free Society*, London: Institute of Economic Affairs.

Seltzer, J.A. (1991), 'Relationships between fathers and children who live apart: the father's role after separation', *Journal of Marriage and the Family*, 53: 79–101.

Sex Education Forum (1993), *Changes to Sex Education Provision*, Sex Education Forum, London: National Children's Bureau.

Sexty, C. (1990), *Women Losing Out: Access to housing in Britain today*, London: Shelter.

Showstack Sassoon, A. (ed.) (1987), *Women and the State*, London: Hutchinson.

Shucksmith, J., Philip, K. *et al.* (1994), 'Between the devil and the deep blue sea: professional educators' attempts to teach about sexuality', paper presented to the British Sociological Association Conference, Preston.

Sinclair, I., Parker, R., Leat, D. and Williams, J. (1990), *The Kaleidoscope of Care: A preview of research on welfare provisions for elderly people*, London: HMSO.

Siraj-Blatchford, I. (1993), *Race, Gender and the Education of Teachers*, Milton Keynes: Open University Press.

Skinner, C. (1994), 'Negotiation and reciprocity: a framework for understanding separated fathers' definitions of parental responsibility', BA in Social Policy dissertation, University of York.

Skrabanek, P. (1988), 'The debate over mass mammography in Britain: the case against', *British Medical Journal*, 297: 991–2.

Skrabanek, P. and McCormick, J. (1989), *Follies and Fallacies in Medicine*, Glasgow: Tarragon Press.

Sly, F. (1993), 'Women and the labour market', *Employment Gazette* (November): 483–502.

Smart, C. (1989), 'Power and the politics of custody', in C. Smart and S. Sevenhuijsen (eds), *Child Custody and the Politics of Gender*, London: Routledge.

Smith, D.E. (1988), *The Everyday World as Problematic*, Milton Keynes: Open University.

Smith, K. (1989), *Housing Agencies for Elderly Owner Occupiers*, London: SHAC.

Smith, L.T. (1993), 'Maori women, education and the struggles for Mana Wahine', in M. Arnot and K. Weiler (eds), *Feminism and Social Justice in Education*, London: Falmer Press.

Sontag, S. (1978), 'The double standard of ageing', in V. Carver and P. Liddiard (eds), *An Ageing Population*, London: Hodder & Stoughton.

Spelman, E. (1988) *Inessential Women: Problems of exclusion in feminist thought*, Boston: Beakon Press.

Spivak, G. (1986), 'Imperialism and sexual difference', *Oxford Literary Review*, 8, 1–2: 225–40.

SSI/DoH (1991), *Women in Social Services: A neglected resource*, Department of Health and SSI, London: HMSO.

Stacey, J. (1991), 'Promoting normality: Section 28 and the regulation of sexuality', in S. Franklin, C. Lury and J. Stacey (eds), *Off Centre: Feminism and cultural studies*, London: Harper Collins Academic.

Stacey, J. (1993), 'Untangling feminist theory', in D. Richardson and V. Robinson (eds), *Introducing Women's Studies*, Basingstoke: Macmillan.

Stanley, L. (ed.) (1991), *Feminist Praxis: Research, theory and epistemology in feminist sociology*, London: Routledge.

Stark, E. and Flitcraft, A. (1988), 'Women and children at risk: a feminist perspective on child abuse', *International Journal of Health Services*, 18, 1: 97–118.

Steedman, C. (1994), 'Bimbos from hell', *Social History*, 19, 1: 57–67.

Steer, P. (1993), 'Rituals in ante-natal care: do we need them?', *British Medical Journal*, 307: 697–8.

Stewart, J., Lewis, N., *et al.* (1992), *Accountability to the Public*, London: European Policy Forum for British and European Market Studies.

Strube, M.J. (1988), 'The decision to leave an abusive relationship: empirical evidence and theoretical issues', *Psychological Bulletin*, 104, 2: 236–50.

Studd, J. (1988), cited by Liz Hodgkinson in 'Elixir of youth?', *Women's Journal* (September): 65–72.

Summers, D. (1991), 'No room for new faces at the top', *Financial Times*, 7 May.

Swift, M. *et al.* (1991), 'Incidence of cancers in 161 familiar affected by ataxia – Tel angiectasia', *The New England Journal of Medicine*, 325, 26: 1831–6.

Sykes, R. (1994), 'Elderly women's housing needs', in R. Gilroy and R. Woods (eds), *Housing Women*, London: Routledge.

Symon, P. (1990), 'Marital breakdown, gender and home ownership: the owner-occupied home in separation and divorce', in P. Symon (ed.), *Housing and Divorce*, Glasgow: Centre for Housing Research.

Taylor-Gooby, P. (1994), 'Postmodernism and social policy: a great leap backwards', *Journal of Social Policy*, 23, 3: 385–404.

Tester, S. (1992), *Common Knowledge: A coordinated approach to information-giving*, London: Centre for Policy on Ageing.

Tester, S. (1994), 'Implications of subsidiarity for the care of older people in Germany', *Social Policy and Administration*, 28, 3: 251–62.

Tester, S. (1995), *Community Care for Older People: A comparative perspective*, Basingstoke: Macmillan.

The Lancet (1993), Editorial, 342, 8866: 251–2.

Thomas, M.D. and Sillen, S. (1976), *Racism and Psychiatry*, New Jersey: Citadel Press.

Thomson, R. and Scott, S. (1990a), *Researching Sexuality in the Light of AIDS*, London: Tufnel Press.

Thomson, R. and Scott, S. (1990b), *Learning about Sex*, London: Tufnel Press.

Thornton, R. (1990), *The New Homeless*, London: SHAC.

Thorogood, N. (1992), 'Private medicine: "you pay your money and you gets treatment" ', *Sociology of Health and Illness*, 14, 1: 23–38.

Titmuss, R.M. (1958), 'The social division of welfare: some reflections on the search for equity', in R.M. Titmuss (ed.), *Essays on the Welfare State*, London: Unwin.

Titmuss, R.M. (1968), *Commitment to Welfare*, London: Allen & Unwin.

Todd, J.E. (1990), *Care in Private Homes, Office of Population Censuses and Surveys*, London: HMSO.

Tomlinson, J. (1990), *Hayek and the Market*, London: Pluto Press.

Townsend, P. (1962), *The Last Refuge*, London: Routledge & Kegan Paul.

Townsend, P. (1970), 'The objectives of the new local social service', in P. Townsend, A. Sinfield, B. Kahan, P. Mittler, H. Rose, M. Meacher, J. Agate, T. Lynes and D. Bull (eds), *The Fifth Social Service: Nine Fabian essays*, London: Fabian Society.

Townsend, P. (1986), 'Ageism and social policy', in C. Phillipson and A. Walker (eds), *Ageing and Social Policy*, Aldershot: Gower.

Townsend, P. and Davidson, N. (eds) (1992), 'The Black Report', in *Inequalities in Health*, Harmondsworth: Penguin.

Truman, C. (1992), 'Demographic change and "new opportunities for woman": the case of employers' career break schemes', in S. Arber and N. Gilbert (eds), *Women and Working Lives: Division and change*, London: Macmillan.

Tunissen, C. and Knapen, M. (1991), 'The Netherlands', in R. Kraan *et al.*, *Care for the Elderly: Significant innovations in three European countries*, Frankfurt-on-Main: Campus Verlag.

Twigg, J. (ed.) (1992), *Carers: Research and practice*, London: HMSO.

Twigg, J. and Atkin, K. (1993), *Carers Perceived: Policy and practice in informal care*, Buckingham: Open University Press.

Ungerson, C. (1983), 'Women and caring: skills, tasks and taboos', in D. Gamarnikov, D. Morgan, J. Purvis and D. Taylorson (eds), *The Public and the Private*, London: Heinemann.

Ungerson, C. (ed.) (1985), *Women and Social Policy: A reader*, Macmillan Women in Society Series, London: Macmillan.

Ungerson, C. (1987), *Policy is Personal: Sex, gender and informal care*, London: Tavistock.

Ungerson, C. (1990), 'The language of care: crossing the boundaries', in C. Ungerson (ed.), *Gender and Caring: Work and welfare in Britain and Scandinavia*, Hemel Hempstead: Harvester Wheatsheaf.

Ussher, J. (1989), *The Psychology of the Female Body*, London: Routledge.

Volger, C. and Pahl, J. (1993), 'Social and economic change and the organisation of money within marriage', *Work, Employment and Society*, 7, 1: 71–95.

Wagner Committee (1988), *Residential Care: A positive choice*, report of the Independent Review of residential care, NISW, London: HMSO.

Waine, B. (1992), 'Workers as owners: the ideology and practice of personal pensions', *Economy and Society*, 21, 1: 27–44.

Walby, S. (1990a), 'From private to public patriarchy: the periodisation of British history', *Women's Studies International Forum*, 13, 6: 91–104.

Walby, S. (1990b), *Theorizing Patriarchy*, Oxford: Blackwell.

Walentowicz, P. (1990), *Caught in the Act Again*, London: SHAC.

Walker, A. (1992), 'The poor relation: poverty among older women', in C. Glendinning and J. Miller (eds), *Women and Poverty: The 1990s*, Hemel Hempstead: Harvester Wheatsheaf.

Walker, A. (1993), 'A cultural revolution? Shifting the UK's welfare mix in the care of older people', in A. Evers and I. Svetlik (eds), *Balancing Pluralism: New welfare mixes in care for the elderly*, Aldershot: Avebury.

Walker, A., Alber, J. and Guillemard, A.M. (1993), *Older People in Europe: Social and Economic policies*, Brussels, Commission of the European Communities.

Walker, R. and Ahmad, W. (1994), 'Windows of opportunity in rotting frames? Care providers' perspectives on community care and black communities', *Critical Social Policy*, 40: 46–69.

Walker, R., Middleton, S. and Thomas, M. (1994), 'Mothers' attachment to child benefit', *Benefits*, 11: 14–17.

Wallace, M. (1979), *Black Macho and the Myth of Superwoman*, London: John Calder.

Walmsley, J., Reynolds, J., Shakespeare, P. and Woolfe, R. (eds) (1993), *Health, Welfare and Practice: Reflecting on role and relationships*, London: Sage.

Ward, M. (1990), *The Local Government and Housing Act, 1989: A guide to the housing aspects*, Coventry: Institute of Housing.

Warner, N. (1994), *Community Care: Just a fairy tale?*, London: Carers National Association.

Watson, S. (1988), *Accommodating Inequality: Gender and housing*, Sydney: Allen & Unwin.

Watson, S. and Austerberry, H. (1986), *Housing and Homelessness: A feminist perspective*, London: Routledge & Kegan Paul.

Watt, S. and Cook, J. (1989), 'Another expectation unfulfilled: black women and Social Services Departments', in C. Hallett (ed.), *Women and Social Services Departments*, Hemel Hempstead: Harvester Wheatsheaf.

Webb, A. and Wistow, G. (1987), *Social Work, Social Care and Social Planning: The personal social services since Seebohm*, Harlow: Longman.

Webster, B. (1985), 'A women's issue: the impact of local authority cuts', *Local Government Studies*, 11, 2: 19–46.

Wedderburn, D. (1965), *Facts and Theories of the Welfare State*, in R. Miliband and J. Saville (eds), *The Socialist Register*, London: Merlin.

Weiner, G. (1994), *Feminisms in Education*, Milton Keynes: Open University Press.

Wenger, G.C. (1994), *Understanding Support Networks and Community Care: Network assessment for elderly people*, Aldershot: Avebury.

Whelan, R. (1994), *Broken Homes and Battered Children*, Family Education Trust.

Whitting, G. (1992), 'Women and poverty: the European context', in C. Glendinning and J. Millar (eds), *Women and Poverty: The 1990s*, Hemel Hempstead: Harvester Wheatsheaf.

Whyte, J., Deem, R., *et al.*, (1985), *Girl Friendly Schooling*, London: Methuen.

Wilding, P. (1992), 'Social policy in the 1980s: an essay on academic evolution', *Social Policy and Administration*, 26, 2: 107–16.

Wiles, R. (1993), 'Women and private medicine', *Sociology of Health and Illness*, 15, 1: 68–85.

Willetts, D. (1993), *The Family*, Contemporary Papers no. 14, W.H. Smith.

Williams Committee (1967), *Caring for People: Staffing residential homes*, London: Allen & Unwin.

Williams, C.J. (1991), 'Health of the nation: the BMJ view', London: British Medical Journal.

Williams, F. (1987), 'Racism and the discipline of social policy', *Critical Social Policy*, 20: (Autumn) 4–29.

Williams, F. (1989), *Social Policy: A critical introduction*, Cambridge: Polity Press.

Williams, F. (1992), 'Somewhere over the rainbow', in N. Manning and R. Page (eds), *Social Policy Review 4*, Harlow: Longman.

Williams, F. (1993), 'Women and community', in J. Bornat, C. Pereira, D. Pilgrim and F. Williams (eds), *Community Care: A reader*, Basingstoke: Macmillan.

Wilson, A. (1978), *Finding a Voice: Asian women in Britain*, London: Virago.

Wilson, A. (1994), 'Sectoral and occupational change: prospects for women's employment', in R. Lindley (ed.), *Labour Market Structures and Prospects for Women*, Manchester: Equal Opportunities Commission.

Wilson, E. (1977), *Women and the Welfare State*, London: Tavistock.

Wilson, E. (1980), 'Feminism and social work', in R. Bailey and M. Brake (eds), *Radical Social Work and Practice*, London: Arnold.

Wilson, G. (1994), 'Co-production and self-care: new approaches to managing community care services for older people', *Social Policy and Administration*, 28, 3: 236–50.

Wilson, M. and Daly, M. (1992), 'Till death us do part', in J. Radford and D. Russell (eds), *Femicide: The politics of woman killing*, Buckingham: Open University Press.

Women's Aid Federation England (WAFE) (1993), *Briefing Papers*, Bristol: WAFE.

Yates, L. (1993), 'Feminism and Australian state policy: some questions for the 1990s', in M. Arnot and K. Weiler (eds), *Feminism and Social Justice in Education*, London: Falmer Press.

Young, I. (1990), *Justice and the Politics of Difference*, Princeton: Princeton University Press.

Zabalza, A. and Tzannatos, Z. (1985), *Women and Equal Pay: The effects of legislation on female employment and wages*, Cambridge: Cambridge University Press.

Zack-Williams, T. and Dennis, F. (1994), 'Ethnicity and gender in access education: some comments on the experiences of African-Caribbean men within the academy', paper presented at the forty-third Annual Conference of the British Sociological Association, held at the University of Central Lancashire, Preston, 28–31 March.

Index

Index